Contents

About the author

Jenny Temple MA, DMS, BSc, RN qualified in the mid-1970s and worked in a variety of settings in London and the South West before moving into nurse education, firstly with the NHS and latterly at Plymouth University. She has a wealth of experience at all educational levels and as an External Examiner.

Jenny has maintained her clinical nursing links with orthopaedics and has research and publications in this area, including a Cochrane Database Review. However, the focus of much of her teaching has been management theory; she believes that good leadership and quality assurance are more than just form-filling and are the key to effective organisational function at all levels. This book is the culmination of her thoughts, which she hopes you will enjoy.

Becoming a Registered Nurse

Making the Transition to Practice

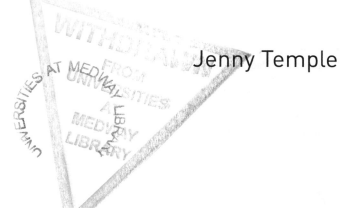

Jenny Temple

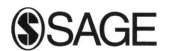 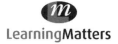

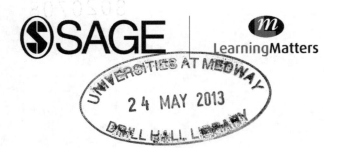

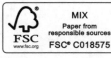

Learning Matters
An imprint of SAGE Publications Ltd
1 Oliver's Yard
55 City Road
London EC1Y 1SP

SAGE Publications Inc.
2455 Teller Road
Thousand Oaks, California 91320

SAGE Publications India Pvt Ltd
B 1/I 1 Mohan Cooperative Industrial Area
Mathura Road
New Delhi 110 044

SAGE Publications Asia-Pacific Pte Ltd
3 Church Street
#10-04 Samsung Hub
Singapore 049483

Editor: Becky Taylor
Development editor: Caroline Sheldrick
Production controller: Chris Marke
Project management: Swales & Willis Ltd,
    Exeter, Devon
Marketing manager: Tamara Navaratnam
Cover design: Wendy Scott
Typeset by: Swales & Willis Ltd, Exeter, Devon
Printed by: MPG Books Group, Bodmin, Cornwall

First published 2012

Library of Congress Control Number: 2012938958

British Library Cataloguing in Publication data

A catalogue record for this book is available from
the British Library

ISBN 978 1 44625 703 6
ISBN 978 0 85725 931 8 (pbk)

Foreword

The transition from novice nurse to expert is a long journey as the seminal work of Patricia Benner (1982) has taught us. Benner proposed that there were five levels of transition, beginning with the novice stage moving through the stages of advanced beginner, competent and proficient to finally reaching expert levels. In this book, Jenny Temple gives some excellent guidance for nursing students on how to make that transition as a novice nurse from the final year to confidently working as a fully qualified practitioner.

There are chapters that will take you through understanding how you become an independent practitioner away from the apron-strings of a mentor. Making decisions and dealing with leadership issues will be skills that you have studied and observed, but will be expected to carry out on your own. In the text, Jenny provides you with examples and scenarios to help consolidate that knowledge and experience to be re-shaped into your new professional role.

You will find the book revisits some of the topics in other texts in the Transforming Nursing Practice series and brings them together so that you can see how these topics, such as assessing risks, taking responsibility for the deteriorating patient and juggling competing demands can be incorporated into your new role.

In the world we inhabit today, there are high public expectations and nurses need to be prepared to deal with patients' complaints to ensure high quality care is provided. Consequently, there is also a chapter in this book which gives guidance on this sensitive area. The final chapter gives you a chance to reflect on what you want for the future: your own personal and professional development. There are many potential pathways that you might want to take to achieve the stages of competence, outlined by Benner, to becoming an expert, and reading this book is one of the first steps.

Shirley Bach
Series Editor

Acknowledgements

The author and publisher would like to thank the following for permission to reproduce copyright material:

Marquis, B and Huston, C (2006) Comparing transactional and transformational leaders, in *Leadership Roles and Management Functions in Nursing; Theory and Application*. Copyright © Lippincott, Williams and Wilkins, for material in Table 4.2, Transactional and transformational leadership.

Maslow, A (1970) *Motivation and Personality*, 2nd edition, Harper & Row, New York. Copyright © Lippincott, Williams and Wilkins, for material in Figure 3.1, Maslow's hierarchy of needs.

Every effort has been made to trace all copyright holders within the book, but if any have been inadvertently overlooked the publisher will be pleased to make the necessary arrangements at the first opportunity.

Introduction

Who is this book for?

Becoming a Registered Nurse is specifically written for the final-year nursing student and those recently registered. It examines in practical detail the issues you will face in managing both yourself and others at work as you complete your pre-registration education and your first year or two of post-qualified employment.

Whatever their field of nursing, all newly registered nurses have to deal with management, leadership and complex care issues which they will not have encountered as students. Through the use of detailed scenarios, these issues are unfolded and you are guided through the theory and practice of nursing in today's health service. It is hoped this book will help you complete your final year in education with confidence and get off to a flying start in your first role.

Book structure

Chapter 1: Making the most of your final year as a student

This chapter covers the different expectations of you in the final year, including delegating to other staff. The issues and anxieties associated with completing your final year, registration and planning your future career are discussed.

Chapter 2: Becoming an independent practitioner

This chapter builds on the delegation skills introduced in the first chapter, and discusses management styles, good management techniques and how to lead a team effectively.

Chapter 3: Dealing with change

This chapter recognises the need for change in the workplace, how this can be managed effectively and how to manage other staff members as they deal with change.

Chapter 4: Working with staff: your role as a leader

This chapter considers situations where leadership is required and how you can demonstrate leadership traits.

Chapter 5: Taking on a mentorship role

This chapter shows you how to recognise learning opportunities in practice and how teaching works in action, as you move from the role of mentee to that of mentor.

Chapter 6: Risks and decisions

This chapter covers risk assessment, decision-making and managing risks in the clinical environment and the staff management issues involved.

Chapter 7: Nursing the deteriorating patient

This chapter considers how to recognise that a patient is deteriorating and how team work, clinical decision-making and effective communication influence care.

Chapter 8: How to manage competing demands

This chapter deals with handling competing pressures in work, managing your own workload and prioritising effectively.

Chapter 9: What if someone wants to make a complaint?

This chapter considers how and why complaints develop and the importance of considering the 'broader picture' in patient care.

Chapter 10: Developing your career: is there a perfect route?

This chapter will remind you about your transferable skills, how these can be used in your career development and the factors involved in maintaining your registration.

Requirements for the NMC Standards for Pre-registration Nursing Education and the Essential Skills Clusters

The Nursing and Midwifery Council (NMC) has established standards of competence to be met by applicants to different parts of the register, and these are the standards it considers necessary for safe and effective practice. In addition to the competencies, the NMC has set out specific skills that nursing students must be able to perform at various points of an education programme. These are known as Essential Skills Clusters (ESCs). This book is structured so that it will help you to understand and meet some of the competencies and ESCs required for entry to the NMC register. It also helps you to understand how to bring together your knowledge and skills at the end of your programme in order to evidence and meet the NMC requirements for registration. The relevant competencies and ESCs are presented at the start of each chapter so that you can clearly see which ones the chapter addresses. The standards are generic ones that all nursing students, irrespective of their field, must achieve, as the material is not field-specific.

This book includes the latest standards for 2010 onwards, taken from *Standards for Pre-registration Nursing Education* (NMC, 2010).

Learning features

Scenarios

Each chapter presents the material in the form of narrative scenarios from various practice settings, which you can easily relate to. These stories are followed by discussion which includes the theory behind good practice. Theory on management, leadership and nursing practice is used to explain why and how certain activities should occur.

The scenarios are set in different fields of nursing practice but the NMC domains and competencies used are always the generic standards that all nurses must meet. The ESC standards identified are those applied at the level of entry to the register. The scenarios, written in such a way as to place you at the centre of the action, are designed to help you consider yourself in the situation. Regardless of the field of practice in which the scenario is set, the problem for discussion is generic and common to all places of work.

Activities

Throughout the book you will find activities that will help you to make sense of, and learn about, the material being presented.

Some activities ask you to reflect on aspects of practice, or your experience of it, or the people or situations you encounter. Reflection is an essential skill in nursing, and it helps you to understand the world around you and often to identify how things might be improved. Other activities will help you develop key skills such as your ability to think critically about a topic in order to challenge received wisdom, or your ability to research a topic and find appropriate information and evidence, and to be able to make decisions using that evidence in situations that are often difficult and time-pressured. Lastly, some ask you to consider your communication skills, to help develop these.

All the activities require you to take a break from reading the text, think through the issues presented and carry out some independent study, possibly using the internet. Where appropriate, sample answers are presented at the end of each chapter, and these will help you to understand more fully your own reflections and independent study.

You might want to think about completing these activities as part of your personal development plan or link them to aspects of the *Knowledge and Skills Framework* (NHS, 2004).

Further reading and useful websites

Each chapter ends with advice on resources for further study; these are frequently websites, where you can learn more about the chapter topic or another one just touched on in context.

And finally . . .

I really do hope that this book helps you understand how to make the transition from student to registered nurse, and gives you the confidence to succeed in your final year or first nursing role. An important part of this transition is understanding how to behave as a 'leader' and role model in all aspects of your nursing care. This is even more important in nursing today, as expectations of nurses grow in response to the increasingly complex care environments that we face. I firmly believe that all registered nurses, even if they are only newly qualified, have to display leadership skills within a rapidly changing healthcare environment, and that doing so is essential to the role of a nurse. Enjoy the book, and good luck in your final year or first post!

Chapter 1
Making the most of your final year as a student

Introduction

Your final year as a nursing student will feel different to previous years. You may have feelings of both nervousness about what will be expected of you this year, and some sadness, perhaps, that your final year is coming to an end. Many students report feeling under a lot of pressure in this final year, from passing assessments through to the increased autonomy and responsibility expected in their final practice learning experiences, which can include some delegating to other staff. There is no doubt that the final year can be tough. You will be expected to be operating at a higher level now, both in your academic work, where you will be expected to be thinking critically and learning independently, and in practice, where you will be expected to demonstrate the ability to be an independent practitioner, a team leader and an effective decision-maker under pressure. But this year is also exciting; now, finally, you can pull together all the knowledge and skills learnt throughout the rest of your course and see it all working in practice. It is natural to feel nervous, but acknowledging that everyone feels this way and learning to appreciate your own strengths and abilities, as well as areas for development, will enable you to succeed in this final year and enjoy it too.

This chapter will use an extended scenario to show what is expected of you in this final year and how to cope with the pressures and demands in order to succeed at it. It will look first at the pressures that you are likely to be feeling and how to cope with them. It will help you to identify your strengths and weaknesses, and consider how to develop your portfolio in your final year. It will explore your final placements or practice learning experiences, what is expected and how to make a success of them. It will also explore the step-up to delegating to other staff that will be part of your final placements. It will touch on planning for your future, which is an important part of your final year, and which will also be explored in more detail in Chapter 10.

Dealing with final-year pressure and anxieties

Scenario

You are a third-year student nurse who has already experienced a range of placements over the last two years, having commenced your nurse training straight after leaving school. In particular, you have spent time with the district nursing team and on two medical care areas, one of which was in a community hospital and the other the stroke unit of a busy district general hospital.

You have been told that your next placement will be in the intensive care unit (ICU) and the final one in a surgical ward. This has made you very anxious as you feel unprepared for either of these areas or for what might be expected of you, as you are in your third year. You have heard from colleagues that the ICU has very high standards of care and similar expectations of its students. You are sure that you will be the least competent student that they have ever had and will fail to cope with the pressures. In fact, despite a good range of marks for your academic work and passes in practice, you think you might as well leave now rather than waste everyone's time.

Your flatmates try to reassure you but this doesn't really help, although you agree not to resign straight away.

Activity 1.1   *Decision-making*

Faced with the situation in this scenario, what do you think you should do?

An outline answer is provided at the end of the chapter.

It is clear that you need to talk to someone about the situation and that your flatmates, although supportive, lack any real idea of what to do. Every university student has an allocated personal tutor and in nursing this is usually someone on the same part of the NMC register (NMC, 2008a). You may feel that this person will not understand the situation but your personal tutor will have considerable experience with student issues and will be able to discuss your options.

It is important that you start to consider tutors or senior clinical staff as colleagues who can assist you, perhaps as a sounding board for ideas, rather than simply as your assessors. In the world of work the function of clinical supervision (NHSME, 1993, in NMC, 2008a) can support staff to work through issues.

You might also think of talking to your parents or 'significant others' as they too may be able to empathise with you and suggest support mechanisms. Here again you are shifting your relationship with adults away from adult–child towards adult–adult, so that you ultimately make your own decisions; this is a concept taken from Berne's (1964) ideas of transactional analysis.

Clearly, it will help to contact the placement and ask to talk about your concerns with a mentor (NMC, 2008a) or someone senior. It may be that your concerns are typical of students being placed on ICU, particularly late in their programme. You need to take control of your learning experiences and develop in a proactive way

Using others to help you address your anxieties

Scenario

You ring the ICU and ask to speak to one of the mentors and are given the dates and times of your shifts. Unfortunately, it was apparently very busy on the unit and the staff nurse couldn't talk to you at length. Of course this has made you even more concerned and you are 'forced' to book an appointment with your personal tutor. You have never asked to meet your tutor before, and have previously always responded to his e-mail request for an appointment at the end of each placement. It is clear that this situation is different, as you are still considering resigning and think of yourself as a failure. Your tutor agrees to see you in a couple of days' time.

Activity 1.2   *Reflection*

What are your own anxieties as you approach the end of your programme? Make a private list of the main things which concern you at this stage. Thinking about your own anxieties as you move towards the end of your pre-registration period will help you prepare for future situations, such as applying for a job.

As this is a personal reflection, no outline answer is supplied.

It is apparent that up to now you have not taken the lead in requesting help, but ownership of a problem and the ability to manage it are signs of maturity. You need to think through why you feel that resignation is your only option, particularly towards the end of your programme.

Once you qualify you will work with learners who themselves express concerns about continuing with a programme of learning. As a true mentor, helping individuals work through issues, such as their suitability for a programme, stress, anxiety or ill health can be a real asset to a student, even if only by referring them to specialist support. Your university or practice base will often have a list of helpful contacts.

Scenario

Your tutor, John, is very welcoming and instead of a designated half-hour tutorial, he offers you a cup of tea, as he's just put the kettle on, and he says that he is free to talk for as long as it takes. He asks you to explain why you wanted to meet and how he can help, but firstly asks you to recap your placements to date and your academic achievements, as he doesn't have your file. You tell him about your marks and your range of placements and then your fears for the final year's placements. All of this comes out as a rushed jumble of words and you know that you haven't made a good impression. You have probably only compounded your own worst fears! So John asks you to take a deep breath and start again, this time much slower and with more detail.

Activity 1.3   *Communication*

Why do you think John wants to know what has been happening to you on the programme to date? What is the purpose of this questioning within the role of tutor?

An outline answer is provided at the end of the chapter.

Getting to the root of a problem can be very difficult, particularly when individuals feel that they are alone and that no one else can have experienced the same concerns. By getting you to repeat, slowly, your concerns, John is asking you to take some control of the problem. He is not belittling your concerns but trying to get you to be in charge. John asks you to talk about issues that you have achieved already, thus providing you with some positive reinforcement. This is a way of starting the conversation in a structured way, and allows you to reflect on your experiences, in particular the successes.

Scenario

You start again, this time more calmly, and find yourself explaining all about how you have enjoyed the community placements with the opportunity to follow some patients' care over several weeks. You are fearful that you will now not have the clinical skills necessary for ICU work or be able to cope with the speed of throughput on a busy surgical ward. You explain that, as you understand the need for this type of placement on the programme and you won't be able to cope, you might as well resign now!

John then asks you about what you have enjoyed during the previous placements, and why. You start to talk about what it was like working on the stroke unit and why you found it so enjoyable; in brief, it was the continuity of care and the feeling that you were really making

continued . . .

a difference to someone's life. The tutor asks you again whether your mentor would think the care you gave was one of your strengths, and reluctantly you agree.

Then you start to describe how it wasn't really your care that worked but the effective communication between the members of the multidisciplinary team and between the hospital and community staff. You don't acknowledge your part in the effective communication until questioned by your tutor, who reminds you about a comment from your mentor on one of the practice summative assessment documents. At last you acknowledge that, yes, you have been complimented on your effective communication skills, both verbal and non-verbal.

Activity 1.4   *Communication*

Why do you think communication skills are so important and will be needed in the months leading to your registration?

An outline answer is provided at the end of the chapter.

Communication

You will need to demonstrate written communication through your portfolio and CV, which you will be expected to present to future employers in job applications. You may then have to build on these written skills in a verbal interview, which may build in further written, mathematical or psychometric tests. (There are more details on applying for other posts in Chapter 10.)

If you are particularly proud of something that has taken place during your programme, then you should bring this to the attention of future employers. For instance, you may have received an excellent grade for an indepth study of a particular patient which is directly relevant to the post for which you are applying. Or you might have developed a health promotion display and influenced the public or been very active as your cohort representative. These sorts of activities provide 'added value' when competing for jobs with others of your cohort.

When you apply for a job towards the end of your pre-registration programme, you may have your first proper interview or it may be many years since your last one, so don't feel shy about improving your oral or writing skills. As a student, writing critically and professionally about a placement or member of staff is challenging, but a skill that has to be developed because it requires you to take the lead, rather than respond to a set academic question (see Chapters 6 and 7).

Many leadership theorists have noted the importance of appraising staff and most organisations undertake this for their staff annually, as it is designed to enhance motivation. This is usually undertaken in a top-down format, with staff appraised by their line manager. (Leadership styles will be covered in Chapter 4.)

Communication skills are also going to appear in your clinical activities; in particular, you will be expected to participate in staff–client interactions, such as patient handover. Trained nursing staff do not expect students to know everything and they must be open to questions. Nobody should ever be discouraged from asking questions; however, as a third-year student you will be expected to respond to routine patient requests or questions and also know when it is appropriate to ask for help. The routine elements make up the transferable skills and John in the scenario asked about your previous placements to make you aware of what you do know. In the next scene, he asks whether you have ever tried to identify your strengths, the skills that you might use in a variety of settings. In response you state that you've only really thought about your weaknesses and not your strengths and so he suggests that you try to carry out a SWOT analysis on yourself.

Identifying your strengths and weaknesses

A SWOT analysis is a tool used by individuals or organisations to consider their options. The concept of a SWOT analysis comes from marketing (**rapidbi.com**), where a company would consider its options. SWOT stands for strengths, weaknesses, opportunities and threats. Strengths and weaknesses are internal to an organisation; opportunities and threats are external influences on the organisation. As individuals we too can undertake a SWOT analysis, particularly in regard to a set of circumstances or a certain event.

Scenario

John suggests a SWOT analysis with regard to your practice progress on the programme in the meeting, and you produce the following:

Strengths (internal): *I have passed all practice assignments to date and I have experienced both community and hospital placements.*

Weaknesses (internal): *I am not good at drug calculations or asking patients about intimate issues.*

Opportunities (external): *I want to carry out one-to-one care on medical patients, who have intensive nursing needs, and also to learn about intravenous fluid management.*

Threats (external): *I think that staff will expect me to give patient handovers confidently as I am a third-year student, because other students are able to do so, but I don't feel I can.*

As you talk further, John encourages you to reflect on what you have learnt in all your practice areas and what experiences in the medical wards might be useful elsewhere. You had never thought of doing any reflections outside of those required for assignments and certainly hadn't thought that it might be helpful in dealing with anxieties. The tutor then asks if you had ever admitted or assessed a patient, and you happily confirm that staff on the stroke unit had supervised and enabled you to admit several patients safely. He suggests

continued . . .

that the skills, which you were pleased to talk about, suggested an ability that might well be useful on the surgical ward. The patients may have different needs, but a structured approach to planning care would also be usable in the surgical ward. You have to admit that the similarities now seem apparent and maybe it wouldn't be such a scary experience after all. John has helped you put the threats in the context of all the other elements of the SWOT analysis.

As the tutorial seems to be reaching a natural closure you start to leave, but somewhat alarmingly, John asks you about your thoughts for the future once you have qualified and registered. He then goes on to talk about the importance of planning ahead, considering well in advance how you might 'sell yourself'. You go away from the meeting feeling much more reassured about the placements, but a bit puzzled by the comments on forward planning.

Activity 1.5   *Evidence-based practice and research*

Reflection is a powerful tool for helping us make sense of experiences and can help when building a portfolio or application form. Models of reflection such as those of John's or Gibbs (Tate and Sills, 2004) structure your thought process, often in a cyclical manner. Revisit the theory on reflection and the model that you find most helpful.

As this is a personal activity, no outline answer is supplied.

Using your strengths in the future

The tutor in the scenario introduced the concept of transferable skills; the Department of Health has recognised the importance of these through the Knowledge and Skills Framework (KSF: NHS, 2004). This is used by staff at all levels in the NHS to consider the comparable skills in a range of posts. In many organisations it is apparent that there are key skills – one such being communication – which are vital in many posts. The KSF has tried to recognise the levels of these skills across a range of posts, which would not normally be seen as comparable. For instance, the communication skills of the ward receptionist might need to be at the same level as a pathology unit worker, even though these skills might actually be used in different ways. The venepuncturist may have higher-level skills than the staff nurse or junior doctor in the area of venepuncture, yet may function at a lower level in other areas. The range of attributes within an individual's KSF can then be used to identify areas of personal growth or possibly pay grade.

The NHS has identified the types of skills it expects to find in individuals carrying out certain posts or in those applying for work. As a third-year student you can compare your own range of skills to those expected of a staff nurse and identify where you need to develop.

Thus, returning to the scenario, when you write your learning contract with your ICU mentor (and subsequently your surgical unit mentor), you can add items specific to you. These are areas you wish to develop beyond your assessment document, as well as items specific to the placement. For instance, your practice assessment may expect you to administer oral drugs safely under supervision but your own SWOT analysis identifies a need to boost your knowledge of medications. The ICU staff also expect you to be able to carry out an ECG, a skill you have never undertaken before; so you have a lot to learn. In the few days preceding your ICU placement you decide to tidy up your portfolio, to make a better impression, as you realise your ongoing achievement records (OARs) document looks better than anything else.

Activity 1.6   *Critical thinking*

Take time to revisit a copy of your portfolio or OARs document, to look at how you developed over the pre-registration programme. Use it to consider your own strengths and weaknesses. It is often very helpful to look back over a past piece of work and see how we have developed or where weaknesses are still apparent.

As this is a personal activity, no outline answer is supplied.

Your portfolio is an important asset in applying for a job and may also be required by the NMC, as it has the power to request, randomly, portfolios of nurses applying for annual re-registration. The portfolio should be kept up to date as it indicates your commitment to lifelong learning and currency of practice (NMC, 2008b).

Re-reading your OARs document for all the placements over the last two years should make you think about your strengths. It also shows that you have tackled some weaknesses that mentors have brought to your attention and suddenly you feel more confident about the future. Again, you realise that actually you are reflecting on your own past performance and can recognise where you have needed to develop.

The OARs document has been a requirement of the NMC (2010) to show how a student's practice has progressed over the duration of the training programme and for use by the sign-off mentor to use at the end of the final placement. The mentoring role will be discussed more in Chapter 5. But the significance of the final placement mentor (the sign-off mentor) is in preventing any students who are incapable of functioning as a registered nurse in practice being allowed on to the register. It also means that the practice areas as well as the academic base have shared responsibility for those accessing the register for the first time. It may also be used by a personal tutor to assist when writing a reference as your tutor is likely only to have a second-hand view of your practice capabilities. By studying the mentor comments your tutor can add to his or her understanding of your skills beyond the classroom or tutorial.

Dealing with a challenging final-year placement

The wearing of a uniform such as scrubs to reduce cross-infection risks will be discussed in Chapter 6; patients in ICU are immune-compromised by nature of their health status and the invasive monitoring that is used.

Understanding medical staff training

Although you may be familiar with the nursing hierarchy in a hospital, you may not know how medical staff progress through their training. Medical students train for five years and may carry out limited clinical patient activity, and on completion of their degree are pre-registration house officers. In the next two foundation years they are allocated to a series of clinical posts in rotation, and carry the title F1 doctor (with provisional registration) and progress to F2 with full General Medical Council registration (General Medical Council, 2012). Registrar, senior registrar and consultant posts reflect inpatient specialist work whereas others may choose to become general practitioners.

There is a considerable amount of anecdotal evidence indicating the significant role that experienced nursing staff have in the clinical development of junior doctors. However, even as a third-year student nurse, you may well have had as wide a clinical experience as any medical student, even if your knowledge base is different.

The sharing of learning in practice is being advocated and explained through activities such as interprofessional teaching (NMC, 2008b). It has become apparent that working together as students and understanding the differing roles of professionals will help to cement good working relationships once qualified. An understanding of one another's roles and responsibilities as well as good professional regard is the foundation of seamless patient care.

Managing your learning

Scenario

Sally laughs at the doctor's remark, and you feel that it is all right to ask how long it took to feel more comfortable in the unit, and whether you will ever know what is going on. Sally is very reassuring and says that she is already impressed by your interest in the patients' treatments and willingness to help where possible. You can't believe she is really talking about you, but nevertheless go back to the unit a little calmer.

At the end of the shift Sally asks you to write your learning contract and to focus beyond your assessment document and more on what you want to learn. This is a different approach from that of any previous mentor but it makes you think about your SWOT analysis and your transferable skills. You remember being told at some point in the last two years that as an adult learner you should be setting your own objectives and building on existing skills.

Learning contracts are often developed and recorded as part of a formal programme of education, but they can be much more informal. You mention that you are curious about what the physiotherapist is doing to a patient's chest. Sally suggests you spend the next available morning with the physiotherapist, Julie, and learn more about her role in ICU.

As her own physiotherapy student has not started the placement yet, you work with Julie the following day. She explains about artificial ventilation and the role of physiotherapy and encourages you to listen to the patient's chest sounds. When you next meet Sally, she asks you what you have learnt and how this will help with nursing care. As you talk about the day, you recognise that you are reflecting on what occurred, communicating effectively about what you have learnt and thus providing evidence for your portfolio. You recognise that you have gathered evidence on your abilities without thinking about meeting a particular learning requirement, which is different from any previous placement.

A few days later Sally sits down with you and together you review your learning contract. By looking at your learning needs first and then the practice assessment document, you are surprised to find that almost everything is covered. When you talk about this, you realise that you have thought over your concerns and written them into the learning contact and that they reflect the expected challenges to a third-year student. Despite a different range of placements to your peers, you have arrived at a similar developmental point in the programme. As the placement progresses you add in to the learning contract your concerns about delegation to others. You admit to Sally that you are always happy being told what to do and never mind helping out, but that you find it very daunting to ask a colleague, whether junior or senior, to help you: you'd rather struggle alone!

Activity 1.7   *Team working*

Try to think of situations when you were delegated to undertake an activity, for instance collecting medication or admitting a patient. How did this delegation make you feel? Could it have been handled better, and what can you learn from this?

An outline answer is provided at the end of the chapter.

Delegation or dumping: getting it right

One of the most commonly felt problems for a 'delegatee' is that once the activity is completed the 'delegator' does not ask how the activity went. In this way the person who undertook the activity may feel put upon and it is perceived not as delegation but rather as being 'dumped' with an unpleasant activity (NMC, 2008b). As many junior staff feel that they are frequently 'dumped on' with menial or tedious tasks, it is difficult for them to learn how to delegate. To delegate means to make effective use of resources: people and time are as much a resource as equipment or money. So if you are the skilled resource and the task can be undertaken by a less skilled person effectively, then this task should be delegated. As a student you may also delegate tasks upwards, to senior staff (if you don't have the knowledge or skills to carry out the task, e.g. intravenous drug administration). However, the important difference between delegation and dumping is that after delegation there must be feedback and acknowledgment.

As a student taking charge of a group of patients, your mentor will be aware of when and how the medicine round will be undertaken and that you cannot do it alone. So if you delegate this activity to your mentor, as will be expected, you must ask your mentor to undertake it and you will expect some feedback on completion. If you tell a junior colleague to clean up a soiled patient, alone, she or he may feel dumped on and resentful; your colleague will wonder why you cannot help, unless you explain what you will be doing concurrently and that you will assist when free.

Meeting your requirements for entry to the register

Scenario

At the midpoint in the placement you undertake your formative practice assessment and Sally points out that you are still not meeting your own target of delegation. However, she is otherwise pleased with your performance and feels that you will successfully complete your penultimate summative assessment in practice. You think back to the meeting with John and how you so nearly resigned, and are so glad that you didn't.

continued . . .

In the final week of your ICU placement a new healthcare assistant (HCA) starts on ICU and Sally asks you to orient her to the building. As the morning progresses you realise that you have learnt much in a short space of time and that you are using skills from this placement and previous ones.

Sally completes your summative practice assessment later that day and compliments you on your handling of the situation with the HCA, as well as the patient care. She even comments that the unit's matron has wondered whether you have thought of ICU-type work as a career. You weren't even aware that the matron knew who you were, but a good manager is in tune with her team. On the final shift in ICU you realise how much you have learnt and, perhaps even more importantly, what you already knew and that you are actually now looking forward to the surgical placement.

Helping other staff and students to learn is a key to a successful working environment and is covered in Chapter 5. One of the requirements of the NMC *Code of Conduct* (2008b) is to assist with the education and support of colleagues and it is thus a requirement of all registered nurses. It is also very rewarding to help others gain skills: good managers and teachers recognise the benefit of an educated workforce.

Planning for a successful final placement

Scenario

After a short period in the university and some annual leave you are due to start on Petra ward, the orthopaedic surgical ward. Jules is your sign-off mentor and Joe your buddy mentor and they have asked to meet you to visit the unit preplacement. Jules is an experienced nurse and mentor and explains that she will be supporting you and Joe, who is undertaking his mentorship training.

Jules asks to see your OARs document and both she and Joe carefully read through all the comments from the very beginning. They then ask about your experiences on ICU and what you specifically want to learn on Petra. You are particularly keen to be able to care for a number of patients with minimal supervision and to be able to delegate tasks to other members of the team. Jules explains that you will always be on the same shift as Joe or herself. Jules expects you to learn specific surgical care from Joe, but agrees that you must also start to direct him with regard to patient care needs.

You comment that you will find delegating to Joe very difficult, but he laughs and says that he recognises this as a learning experience for you and he won't be offended.

The sign-off mentor role is recognised as being key to ensuring that only those students who are functioning effectively in practice are allowed to register. The NMC Standards to Support Learning and Assessment in Practice (NMC, 2008a) indicate that the mentor and student should work together at least 40% of the time in direct or indirect supervision. However, they specifically qualify the role of the sign-off mentor as requiring an additional weekly meeting to review progress.

One of the difficulties that students experience towards the end of their programme is trying to visualise or enact the role of a trained professional, without actually working beyond their student capacity. An effective mentor will want to challenge you to delegate tasks, under supervision, and observe your potential for professional growth. In the final stages of your pre-registration programme you need to be able to function, in the main, as a qualified nurse. However, there are clearly items which you cannot undertake at all and others that must not be undertaken without supervision.

For example, when you and Joe care for a group of patients, he will expect you to organise his workload for him rather than delegating to you. He will know what time to administer medication but may expect you to remind him; in this way you are learning to prioritise and manage your own time but also that of the team. It is likely that at first you may need prompting to delegate, but as your confidence develops you should be able to organise yourself, your team and the patients' needs.

It will become apparent that, if you try to do all the actions yourself, you will fail and that the only way for teams to function effectively is to share the workload. Asking staff to undertake work should never be a way of avoiding doing something yourself: this is unprofessional and unpleasant. It should be a way of using everyone effectively and efficiently.

Other sources of help

Scenario

As you start working on the ward you realise that you do know how to carry out many tasks and that understanding some aspects of surgical nursing, even those that you haven't met before, isn't really that 'foreign'. You spend time following the patient journey and enhance your understanding of pain and fluid management. You also recognise that not only has ICU provided you with skills, but that many of the medications patients receive are familiar from the medical ward placements. In the same way that ICU set up your learning contract, Jules encourages you to write yours and to build on the practice assessment document, for this, your final placement. Jules also arranges for all three of you to get together weekly to meet the NMC (2008a) requirements of the sign-off mentor role and discuss your progress. Both Jules and Joe frequently ask you to reflect on what you have learnt in the preceding week and what you are aiming for. This has had the effect of really making you consider what aspects of care you need to develop, and to recognise that you have made progress with delegation and medicines management. By the midpoint of the placement you have

continued . . .

had a successful formative assessment and have also submitted all your academic assignments, although you are still awaiting the results. Jules then asks you to review the support you have received from Joe and to write some comments for his portfolio.

As the final weeks of the placement pass, you are confidently handing over patient care to colleagues and have eventually been able to ask other students or trained staff to help you as part of your learning process, but are still not able to delegate to an HCA. Jules asks you to think about this problem and at the same time confirms that your summative assessment in practice has been passed, as you have met all the criteria. You look back over the last year and realise that your lack of confidence nine months ago was probably no different from that of anyone in your student cohort. You recognise that this final placement in particular has pulled on all those transferable skills and helped you take the lead in providing patient care, as appropriate. Jules is also pleased with your progress and will be happy to sign off your competence at the end of the placement. She also asks you about the support you have gained from herself and Joe, encouraging you to give a constructive evaluation of the placement. However, she sets you the task of working with Carol, the HCA, on your own tomorrow, to organise the day-case admissions.

You spend an anxious night wondering how you can possibly ask the HCA, who has been on the unit for many years, to undertake any tasks. Your old worries resurface, but Jules has stressed that you are at the expected level of achievement and that she will ensure there are no untoward events. Once on duty you meet Carol to talk about the shift ahead and what is expected of you both; to your surprise, she is happy with the arrangement. She comments that knowing what is expected of you both is helpful and asks what she should do first. You are aware that Carol can't admit the patient who has already arrived, but it is apparent that there is a shortage of laundry, to make up the theatre bedding. So you suggest that Carol finds laundry and makes up the beds whilst you talk to the admission in the day room; Carol willingly agrees. You are very surprised that she has taken instruction from you, but as you had discussed the priorities and she could only do one of them, it is a reasonable arrangement. Once these first activities have been completed you meet Carol again to agree the next tasks; the morning progresses. Carol asks that she have first break, which you had planned to take and so your first instinct is to decline her request. Then you consider why you felt the need to go first and realise that it was just habit and agree to her request. Carol thanks you and returns promptly from her break having met up with her colleagues as planned.

Activity 1.8   *Team working*

Why do you think it was effective to respond to Carol's request?

An outline answer is provided at the end of the chapter.

Planning for your future

Scenario

Jules also asks you about your plans for the future, in particular whether you have a preferred area of work or whether you are happy to take any post as long as it is based in the locality. She also indicates that she will be happy to provide an employer's reference if requested. You have to admit that you are keen to find any kind of qualified nurse work, and recognise that competition for any post will be fierce. Jules acknowledges the problems, but suggests that a post with some allocated preceptorship will be more helpful in the long term. She reminds you that the trust's nursing bank may offer some posts for newly qualified staff. You hadn't thought of working on the nurse bank, as a trained nurse, but had recently joined as an HCA.

On the final day in placement as a student you realise that you have learnt a lot over three years, not just about nursing, but also about yourself and in part you are ready for the next challenge.

Activity 1.9   *Decision-making*

Why can working as an agency nurse or bank nurse within a trust provide useful experiences?

An outline answer is provided at the end of the chapter.

Preceptorship: a golden opportunity

What is the purpose of preceptorship? The NMC (2010, citing Beck and Srivastava, 1991) recognised that staff on qualifying or on changing posts really need a period of time to settle into the role. This was seen as particularly important in up-skilling newly qualified staff and is difficult if the staff appointee is immediately part of the nursing team and expected to carry a normal workload. However, there are considerable costs to the employer in supporting a preceptorship post and so some trusts or employers may not offer it. In a preceptorship post, the qualified nurse is seen as extra to the normal staffing ratio; this allows for both orientation and additional training. It is also likely that an experienced member of staff will provide a degree of mentoring. However, as a registered nurse certain expectations and accountability in the post will apply. Preceptorship posts may include a short period in a supernumerary status or facilitate rotation through a number of different areas within a trust, but will generally include some additional forms of training.

Taking it further

As this book progresses it will help you to consider your role as an independent practitioner (Chapter 2) and how implementing change is a difficult problem for both individuals and organisations. In Chapter 3 change management will be discussed in depth and how this can be made to happen successfully. It will help you write critically and professionally about a placement or member of staff and how to manage risky situations (Chapter 6). It will consider how leadership styles develop (Chapter 4) and how leadership theorists have noted the importance of effectively managing staff. Chapter 5 will talk about moving to a mentoring role with learners and Chapters 7–9 will deal with deteriorating patients, conflicting priorities and complaints. The final section (Chapter 10) will give thought to furthering your career and applying for new jobs.

You are about to change from a student to a registered professional and it is likely that nothing will quite prepare you for the first time someone calls you staff nurse!

Activities: brief outline answers

Activity 1.1

This first activity is designed to help you think through typical situations, so it has both elements of decision-making and reflection. The important issues are that you don't avoid challenges and that you take risks in order to develop personally and professionally.

Activity 1.3

When you reflect on situations in a structured way, you may be able to remove or amend some of the emotional elements associated with difficult events and so communicate more clearly.

Activity 1.4

Even if you can't state why effective communication is so important, you can probably indicate how poor communication leads to a breakdown in effective care. Typically, good communication goes unnoticed; but when it fails, the resultant poor communication quickly leads to problems.

For instance:

1. In accident and emergency the emergency telephone alerts the staff to an incoming casualty: effective communication means that staff are organised and awaiting the casualty in the acute area on arrival by ambulance.
2. If written records don't record the size, shape and treatment regime of a leg ulcer, how will change be recognised?
3. If there is no communication between team members, they might all choose to go to lunch at the same time, leaving no one to care for the clients.

Activity 1.7

If you were asked to undertake a task, how this was approached and then followed up will have influenced the way you feel. If you agreed that you were either the best person for the activity or it had a learning component, then you were probably keener to do the task. But if no one else was available or the task was tedious you were probably less happy and might have felt dumped on.

Activity 1.8

Working as part of a team requires give and take. Colleagues are much more likely to respond to a request from their manager if they believe their own needs are being considered. If you had been unable to grant Carol her request, it would be important to explain why, as this would help to prevent a breakdown in the relationship.

Activity 1.9

If there is an opportunity to work within a local trust, either as an HCA or after registration, then you will raise your profile with that employer, but some trusts may not accept the newly qualified on the nurse bank. It will also help you understand the care areas where you haven't already worked, either as a student or as an HCA, and local policies and procedures. You may also be offered staff development in the form of statutory updates, medicines management training and uniform, but this will vary between trusts.

Working for an agency will give you the opportunity to work outside the NHS and possibly in a range of different NHS trusts.

Any employer has to provide certain requirements for its staff, such as paid leave and mandatory updates, but the work for the bank or agency will be more varied and you may find that you are expected to travel over a wide geographical area.

Further reading and useful websites

For more information on SWOT analysis and other management tools, go to: **rapidbi.com/swot analysis/**

Remind yourself about the NMC Code of Conduct 2008 at: **www.nmc-uk.org/Nurses-and-midwives/The-code**

Remember that one way to maintain lifelong learning is by reading journals such as:

* *Nursing Times;*
* *Nursing Standard;*
* *Journal of Advanced Nursing.*

Chapter 2
Becoming an independent practitioner

NMC Standards for Pre-registration Nursing Education

This chapter will address the following competencies:

Domain 1: Professional values
1. All nurses must practise with confidence according to *The code: Standards of conduct, performance and ethics for nurses and midwives* (NMC 2008), and within other recognised ethical and legal frameworks. They must be able to recognise and address ethical challenges relating to people's choices and decision-making about their care, and act within the law to help them and their families and carers find acceptable solutions.

NMC Essential Skills Clusters

This chapter will address the following ESCs:

Cluster: Care, compassion and communication
1. As partners in the care process, people can trust a newly registered graduate nurse to provide collaborative care based on the highest standards, knowledge and competence.

By entry to register
14. Uses professional support structures to develop self-awareness, challenge own prejudices and enable professional relationships, so that care is delivered without compromise.

Cluster: Organisational aspects of care
11. People can trust the newly registered graduate nurse to safeguard children and adults from vulnerable situations and protect them from harm.

By entry to register
10. Challenges practices which do not safeguard those in need of support and protection.

> ### Chapter aims
>
> After reading this chapter, you will be able to:
>
> - recognise features of good management style;
> - explain the importance of task delegation;
> - describe how to run a successful meeting;
> - identify how assertiveness is important in managing roles within a team.

Introduction

The scenarios in this chapter are set in a mental health unit, but the principles apply in every healthcare setting.

> ### Scenario
>
> You have been fortunate in obtaining a permanent post on the acute admissions unit's Trafalgar ward in your local mental health trust following a period on the preceptorship programme. The rotational nature of the preceptorship programme has meant that you have worked on the ward previously, but many of the staff have also changed in the intervening months. You have been appointed along with Julie, another newly qualified nurse, and you are both starting your first week's proper employment today.
>
> The shift started at 07.30 with handover and report in the ward office. It is clear that the ward is experiencing a considerable amount of change in both staff and clients, as very few of the patients are known to anyone for more than one or two days. Fortunately, besides you and the other new staff nurse on duty, there is the charge nurse and two healthcare assistants (HCAs), so you are hopeful of some orientation time.
>
> Charge nurse John indicates that you should work with the HCA Ann and your colleague with the HCA Maureen, as he is planning to attend a unit management meeting from 09.30 and mentions that both Ann and Maureen are experienced members of the team. John addresses the HCAs and tells them to go and manage breakfast for the clients while he spends time with you and Julie. You hope that this is an orientation period, but you are aware of the lack of trained staff on the 'floor' with the clients. John gives a brief 'hello and welcome to the unit' speech, reminding you both of medication round times and duration of meal breaks and then says that he has paper work to do before the unit meeting.
>
> The medication cupboard keys are handed to you and Julie and you leave the office. All of a sudden you are aware that there is no supernumerary status, no student role, no preceptee role to fall into: you are expected to be a fully functioning, qualified, autonomous practitioner. All the way through your training, personal accountability was stressed, but there

continued . . .

was always the 'safety blanket' of your mentor/supervisor to support your decision-making. Now you feel horribly alone with the reality of personal accountability and unfamiliar working practices.

Accountability

The scenario describes a fairly typical first day. One of the main differences between student and registered status is accountability, so that is the theme of the first activity.

Activity 2.1   *Reflection*

Think about your accountability when you were a student nurse. Who were you accountable to then? Now reflect briefly on what accountability means once you are registered, and there is no mentor to ask about your practice.

An outline answer is provided at the end of the chapter.

Scenario

Julie jolts you out of your thoughts with a request about whether you want to start the medications administration, or should she start them while you meet the clients? Neither of you feel very confident about understanding the ward's routine but recognise the need to hand out medication. As you have only recently finished the preceptorship circuit on the other admissions ward, Nelson, and, as Julie was in outpatients, you draw the 'short straw' for the medication round. You can vaguely recall where the medication was administered and that the clients came to you, rather than you bringing the drugs trolley around to the patients.

Maureen calls to you that the clean medicine pots are kept in the kitchen between rounds and might still be in the dishwasher; you are very aware that time is moving on rapidly and that you are getting behind. In the kitchen it is clear that breakfast is progressing well and you are offered a cup of tea by the housekeeping staff. You face an immediate but small dilemma, aware that accepting a drink will delay you further but also that declining might make you appear aloof from the team. You politely thank the housekeeper but decline and say that you would appreciate a cup later.

In this scenario, the first real conflict of the day has arisen. Establishing yourself as part of the team in a new post can be very difficult and can feel like walking a tightrope: you want to belong, but you know that you are now in a supervisory position. Intrapersonal conflict is defined by Marquis and Huston (2006) as the anguish faced by managers in trying to balance the competing pressures on them from outside forces, such as the requirements from their supervisor or manager, versus the needs of the junior staff or the client group. In the scenario, declining the offered tea has been one solution to the competing pressures that cause interpersonal conflict. In any job and in most organisations there is a managerial hierarchy and thus different levels of authority so that there has to be a compromise between equity of shared team work and supervision or delegation. If you become 'one of the boys' either in work or at a social event outside, it can become very difficult to change roles if you are required to exercise the authority of a supervisory post. Those to whom you wish to delegate work may feel that you have no right, because they see you as a friend or co-worker rather than a junior manager. However, for any team to function, there must be a good working relationship, for which team bonding is important. So, having tea with the HCAs and housekeeping staff will promote team bonding but is at odds with the requirements of the staff nurse role and the needs of the clients, and thus causes interpersonal conflict as you weigh up the situation in order to make the correct decision.

If, on another occasion, you sit and talk with the HCAs and the housekeeping staff about their role within the organisation, their objectives and career plans it is likely that you will find commonalities of purpose. Shared values and goals will mean there is less likelihood of interpersonal conflict or bullying (horizontal violence) within the organisation and thus it will be a happier place to work with better levels of productivity.

Scenario

You undertake the medications administration and fortunately are able to identify safely all the patients against their drug charts and recognise almost all the drugs and their side effects from memory. Overall you feel that you have done this first task effectively and reasonably quickly. You recognise that there haven't been very many drug rounds previous to this one when you have had no form of supervision. As a student you were never alone and on the preceptorship programme an opportunity was often available for you to discuss issues with your mentor when you had concerns.

You see Julie as you leave the clinical room with the prescription charts that need attention, and ask how her work is going. Julie says OK, she thinks that a couple of the clients don't seem to have comprehensive care plans but otherwise she understands their nursing care regimes. Equally supportive, she asks how you got on and you too have a couple of issues but generally feel contented with the way the drug round went. Julie offers to make tea for both of you while you write notes for the medical staff about the prescription charts.

As you enter the ward office, the ward clerk informs you that the charge nurse has already left early for his meeting and that there are some 'to do' notes in the ward diary. When Julie returns with the cups of tea, she has one for the ward clerk as well; you ask what Ann and Maureen are doing. To your surprise, you are told that they have gone for their break in the canteen, something neither you nor Julie were aware of. The ward clerk says that they should be back within half an hour and that they always take their breaks together.

Management styles and delegation

Activity 2.2   *Leadership and management*

What might be the consequences of the absence of the charge nurse and both HCAs in this situation?

An outline answer is provided at the end of the chapter.

In the scenario, you will have identified that there is clearly an issue of professional accountability concerning departure from the ward of all the trained staff and this clearly should never happen. In your practice, as in the scenario, you need to think about working practices, and in particular thinking about staff as a resource. The Working Time Regulations (1998) specify the length of time staff can work between breaks and rest periods, and it may sometimes be difficult to ensure that this legislation is implemented. The rules specify a 20-minute break in any six-hour working period for those over 18 years old and this must not be taken at the end of the shift. What is really important is that staff can have their breaks at suitable times such that their health and well-being are taken into consideration. The evidence from research shows that staff who are rested work better and are less inclined to make errors (Health and Safety Executive, 2006).

This means that it is important to plan for break times when managing a team of workers, to enable both client safety and staff comfort to be addressed. It should also apply to the leader of the team, who must set a good example and act fairly.

In any workplace there must be an effective use of the skills and resources of every member of the team. You don't pay top rates to a very experienced Band 5 nurse on £27,000 to make the tea and clean flower vases. Staff are the most expensive resource in any workplace and must be used efficiently. When the roles and responsibilities of all the team members are known and understood by all, then they can work effectively together to agreed, common goals.

Theory summary: worker productivity

The findings of Adam Smith in the eighteenth century and Frederick Taylor in the early twentieth century illustrated that if employees became specialists they could increase productivity. Adam Smith, in his 1776 book *An Inquiry into the Nature and Causes of the Wealth of Nations* (**www.bbc.co.uk/history/historic_figures/smith_adam.shtml**), indicated that the more expert a worker became, the more he produced and the better the quality of the item. Smith considered the manufacture of iron nails, which had previously been made in entirety by one worker: he found that breaking the nail production into specific stages led to specialisation and increased productivity. This was taken further by Frederick Taylor (Taylorism) in his 1911 publication *Principles of Scientific Management* (**www.mindtools.com/pages/article/newTMM_Taylor.htm**) and was further developed by Henry Ford (Fordism) in the US car production lines of the early twentieth century.

In the 1920s Elton Mayo started to consider whether the workplace had more significance to individuals than purely financial and recognised the social and psychological aspects of employment. In particular, staff work in ways that may not be anticipated by their employer and this reflects social norms and interactions, and function differently when observed – the 'Hawthorne effect'. He concluded that productivity may relate not just to specialisation but to the interactions between workers and their bosses.

Even more recent studies of employee activity show that it is vital for quality control that staff not only have expert skills in producing a component of a product but must see how this fits within the whole product. This concept also developed in the car production line, where it was noted that some companies had much better quality in their final cars. In particular, workers who participated in many or all aspects of car production made better goods than those who only undertook one aspect, such as repeatedly making door panels. The reasoning was that the individuals who made the whole car could visualise the finished product and how they affected its quality. Those who only make door panels, for instance, see no point in ensuring the quality of the door panel, because it is only perceived as a sheet of metal, not as a functioning car.

Using staff in appropriate roles

How does worker productivity in industry relate to nursing? In many ways, division of labour is replicated in nursing with task allocation: the most junior staff do the most menial tasks while those in authority carry out more expert tasks. In nursing during the 1980s there was a positive move away from task allocation to team work, where there is some hierarchical division of labour, and ultimately to primary nursing (Hegyvary, 1982). In primary nursing the trained nurse leads the team of associate nurses considering every aspect of a patient's care, with little division of labour or role demarcation except in the prescriptive nature of the primary nurse's role. Primary nursing was seen to provide high quality of care and high levels of motivation for the nursing staff, as the product outcome was clearly defined. Primary nursing does provide exceptional care, but, unlike car manufacture, patients are not standard items and it proved difficult to maintain.

In the UK primary nursing as a concept was very difficult to implement and as such there has been a move back to team nursing, taking the best aspects of both primary nursing and task allocation. You may understand the UK's interpretation of the primary nurse by the term 'named nurse', the qualified nurse with key responsibility for a patient's care, but leading a team who deliver different aspects of that day-to-day care.

You will also experience task allocation, typically on night duty or in an emergency situation. Then there is no attempt to carry out all aspects of care, but the work is shared appropriately among the team to meet the situational needs.

Let us return to the scenario of your first day on the ward.

Scenario

Eventually the HCAs return to the ward and Ann suggests that it will be OK if you and Julie want to take a break together now that they are back. You are amazed at this suggestion, and reply that this wouldn't be appropriate as there would be no one trained on duty. The 'shrugged shoulder' response and 'Oh well' comment lead you to believe that the lack of trained staff on duty at any time, however brief, might not be an unusual occurrence. You look to Julie for support and she confirms your concerns, by suggesting that you will take your breaks separately, and suggests you go now before starting anything new.

The ward clerk reminds you both of the start time for the therapy sessions and the expected admission and you agree that Julie should lead the therapy session, as it would fit after her break and you will start the admission process, once you return. The morning progresses well and eventually charge nurse John returns from his meeting.

During the early afternoon you decide to express your concerns about the HCAs' approach to break time with John, and in particular that they felt it would be all right for all the trained staff to be absent at the same time. John appears to be amused by the idea of the HCAs managing their time without reference to you or staff nurse Julie, which makes you feel irritated: he is being unprofessional. However, as your irritation is clearly showing in your non-verbal communication, he changes strategy and agrees to talk it through after the late shift has come on duty to relieve you all.

Activity 2.3 — *Communication*

If it really was you in this scenario, would you feel the same? If you have ever been in a similar situation, how did you communicate your feelings and your opinion?

An outline answer is provided at the end of the chapter.

When staff in a position of authority are visibly insecure, it often happens that more junior staff will take advantage of the situation. This is apparent in the scenario above: when charge nurse John is absent the HCAs decide to have their break together. It can be very difficult for newly appointed or newly qualified staff to exert their authority without being seen as 'bossy' or 'jumped up'. We have all heard people say: 'who does she think she is?' The answer is, you are the person responsible. There are a number of sites online where management styles are illustrated, particularly on YouTube.

Management style

It is important to be able to demonstrate authority and assertiveness quickly while acknowledging the importance of team work and showing empathy for junior staff. If the scenario were re-run, it would have been very helpful if charge nurse John had reinforced the position of you and Julie with the HCAs before going to his meeting. He should have outlined the morning's workload for trained and untrained staff and identified that staff nurse Julie and HCA Maureen would go to break together. This would have been much more explicit than just the comment about the trained nurse/HCA pairings, which he suggested was for orientation only. He would have been aware, from his knowledge of the staff, that given the opportunity these two HCAs might take advantage of inexperienced new staff in any way they could.

Working with junior staff, particularly those who see themselves as experienced, can be a delicate balance for any newly qualified staff nurse. As a student you are often seen as the most junior member of the team, yet once qualified and in receipt of a Nursing and Midwifery Council (NMC) PIN number, you are instantly thought to be both experienced and confident, which may feel very alien as you make the role transition. There needs to be a radical rethink in the way colleagues see your role, particularly if you return to a workplace where you are known as a student. It is also important to change your own attitude, meaning that you are no longer 'one of the girls' but have to consider your professional persona.

Effective managers exist at all levels in the workplace. The staff nurse running a team of one or two HCAs and a student is as much a leader in her way as the ward manager and unit manager in theirs. Some would say that the need to lead an effective nursing care team, working directly with clients, must be the cornerstone of effective healthcare organisations.

Activity 2.4   *Team working*

Have you ever been in a situation where you have done a task yourself as you didn't feel able to ask the colleague or family member whose job it was to do it? Think about why this happened.

An outline answer is provided at the end of the chapter.

Scenario

John, Julie and yourself leave the ward after handover and go to the staff room, and after putting a 'do not disturb' notice on the door, John asks you to talk about this morning. Julie is equally as upset as you and starts the conversation with her concerns: she clearly states that she felt undermined by the HCAs, who didn't value her. John asks why she feels like this and Julie explains that indicating that each of the staff nurses should be paired with an 'experienced HCA who is familiar with the ward' suggests that they have more skills than the registered nurse. You comment that, had the HCAs been directed, by John, to work as a team assisting the trained nurse, the situation might not have arisen. You acknowledge that the HCAs are likely to be more familiar with the day-to-day activities and timings of events, but that his attitude firmly led to them feeling in control and able to make their own decisions without reference to Julie or yourself.

continued . . .

John looks surprised at the depth of feeling being displayed by both you and Julie and apologises, admitting that he really hadn't considered how his managerial style would be interpreted. He recognised that he was rushed for time and hadn't really prepared for his meeting so didn't spend a reasonable time welcoming the two new staff members or setting the ground rules.

He agrees to think about his managerial style and speak to the HCAs in private about their attitude to the new staff nurses. He also thanks you both for actually managing so well this morning and also being so honest with him about your concerns. He asks if you think a staff meeting might be helpful. Julie replies that she would rather he spoke privately to the HCAs first and then wait to see what happens; you agree with this approach.

John took two important steps in managing a potentially difficult encounter in this part of the scenario. First, he recognised the importance of prompt action in dealing with any problem and second, he is indicating its importance by convening a private meeting away from the main ward area and putting up a 'do not disturb' sign.

When convening any meeting of importance it is vital that there are minimal interruptions and maximum opportunity for honest and open discussion. At the end of any meeting there should be a stated outcome agreed by all, even if this is only to meet again on a particular day. If there is no agreed outcome, participants will often feel that, although listened to, their feelings are not being taken seriously.

Managing meetings

You will have been to good meetings, where issues were raised and dealt with effectively, and meetings which were a waste of everyone's time. You will be involved in meetings throughout your career, so learn how to organise them well. Mackenzie (1972, cited by La Monica, 1994, pp 288–9) writes at length about the effective use of time: his work is as relevant today as it was then, although we can now add the e-mail or text message as further ways of interrupting the day. His process for managing meetings effectively is as follows.

1. Start on time; give warning only the first time.
2. End on time.
3. Develop an agenda and circulate it to attendees prior to the meeting.
4. Only those needed should attend a meeting.
5. Gather information prior to a meeting; summarise it during the meeting.
6. Stick to the agenda; avoid interruptions; squash side trips around or away from the agenda.
7. Limit the amount of time for the particular agenda; pace the meeting so that the intended outcomes are accomplished.
8. Arrange for a comfortable environment, but not so plush that people would rather be there than elsewhere.
9. Items that involve one-way communication by their nature should be typed and distributed, not verbally announced, as this wastes time.

10. Have a secretary and distribute the minutes within a week from the date of the meeting. Minutes should record the issues and the decisions. Brief reports of the discussion may be included. When minutes are verbatim accounts of the meetings, the secretary wastes time and so do all the readers.

Although John's meeting was not as formal as this, he managed some of the criteria of effectiveness. The meeting was planned and an effective time slot allocated, without interruption in a place of comfort. It was designed to find out what the problem was, to gather information and an outcome was agreed.

Delegation and assertiveness

In order to manage well and delegate effectively, you need to be assertive. This means being clear and polite but firm.

Scenario

The following day you are on a late shift and it is clear that charge nurse John has spoken to the HCAs about yesterday, as they are slightly distant with you when you meet after handover, which was led by John on the early shift. On the ward with the clients the HCAs ask why you reported them for going to break together; you state that you can't talk in front of the clients but will discuss this later with them. You can envisage a difficult and possibly tearful meeting, but know that their behaviour had the potential to affect patient safety.

In the day room you apologise if they feel they were 'reported' and thus subject to some sort of disciplinary action: this had not been either your or Julie's intention. However you stress that their behaviour did leave you and Julie in a difficult situation, which you couldn't allow to be repeated. You briefly explain how their input is very valuable to both you and Julie, but that as newly qualified members of the team and in John's absence you had to be fully aware of what was happening with staff and clients on the ward. HCA Ann states that she didn't think about the implications of her actions when she and Maureen left the ward together as charge nurse John would frequently allow this. You explain that as John was familiar with the ward, he was in a different situation to you and Julie, more confident and less vulnerable.

The HCAs are surprised that you feel vulnerable and also that you apologised for any bad feelings that were potentially developing between you and them, but admit that they can now see how difficult it was for you yesterday. You end the meeting stating that you want to work as an effective team, delivering safe patient care.

It is clear that the various meetings have had the desired effect on all concerned, as charge nurse John now explains better what he wants done before leaving for any meeting and you and staff nurse Julie have been effectively supported by the HCAs. So today is the first time

continued . . .

that you feel the need to exert your authority over one of the HCAs and delegate a task to her, to be done quickly. One of the clients has been violently sick all around his bed space, Ann was about to leave for lunch and you have called her back. You explain that you need her to clean up the area, as no housekeeping staff are available, while you telephone the relatives and talk to the doctor. Ann is not happy with this arrangement and says that it is unfair and not her responsibility. You are insistent but add that if you get your tasks done, you will come and help her. You check that she has protective clothing and access to cleaning equipment before asking her to get on with the task.

This is the first time that you have delegated an unpleasant activity to a colleague and now find that it has been difficult to insist. As a student you would never have asked an HCA to do an unpleasant task, but recognise that as a staff nurse you have to delegate. You know that although you could take the housekeeping role, the HCA can't talk to the doctor or the relatives, and all these activities are of equal importance. Fortunately the doctor visits the ward, by chance, soon afterwards, and you discuss the client's situation. On his departure you make contact with the client's family to discuss the problem briefly. This means that you are free to go to the client's bed space to help Ann. You find her muttering to herself but also cleaning effectively; you ask if there is anything you can do to help. Ann looks surprised but requests that you take the foul laundry, which she has bagged up, to the sluice, which you do. On your return to Ann, with clean laundry as you noticed this was also needed, you ask if she needs further help, but it is clear that other than remake the bed everything is finished. So together you remake the bed and thank Ann for her speedy work before telling her to take her lunch, apologising for the delay.

Good and poor delegation

Good delegation is illustrated in the scenario: the work being delegated is appropriate for the HCA to carry out. The staff nurse has ascertained that the HCA is both competent to undertake the task and that she has the tools to do the job. She also concurrently undertook activities that the HCA couldn't do. It wasn't 'dumped' on the HCA because the staff nurse returned to find out how the situation was progressing and started to help out. At the end of the activity, when all tasks had been completed satisfactorily, the staff nurse thanked the HCA for delaying her lunch break and for assisting with this appropriate but rather unpleasant activity.

Poor delegation occurred earlier in the scenario when the charge nurse gave a perfunctory welcome to the ward to his newly appointed staff nurses, then left to go to a meeting. He over-delegated to the staff nurses, as they were unaware of the ward routines or protocols, but are professionally competent. He delegated improperly to the HCAs, who were led to believe they could organise their own coffee break without discussion with the staff nurses, such that they were making decisions outside their professional boundaries.

Activity 2.5　　　　　　　　　　　　　　　*Leadership and management*

Be honest with yourself: have there been times at work when you delegated a task because it was simply unpleasant? With hindsight, can you justify your actions?

As this activity is based on personal reflection, no outline answer is supplied.

Delegation is frequently a difficult task for newly qualified staff to undertake and needs to be practised to get it right. Marquis and Huston (2006) identify three common errors in delegation that apply to many managers: over-delegation, under-delegation and improper delegation. It is frequently under-delegating that is the problem for newly qualified staff, who may feel that by delegating to others they will be judged as not working hard enough or being bossy. In reality, effective delegation makes best use of resources because it matches the work to the worker, and the hierarchy of most organisations means delegation is invariably downwards.

Over-delegation is less likely for junior staff, but they may work in a situation where too many tasks or objectives are passed to them by their manager. If the manager is trying to develop skills in junior staff he or she may delegate tasks to grow their talents and enhance their experience. In this instance the support and supervision from the manager are necessary, but over-delegation is where excessive tasks are passed on and there is no support. This may occur when the manager fails to use his or her own time wisely and is thus required to carry out multiple tasks concurrently or when the manager feels clinically incompetent.

Staff development and delegation

You need to be aware of the subtle difference between over-delegation and staff development. In staff development, a manager supports a more junior colleague to undertake a task which the manager would normally do. For instance, historically senior managers might have monitored and then purchased items for a ward, but monitoring or stock control is a basic task which can be undertaken by staff without professional registration. However, the signature of the budget-holder on order forms may be required, and this person is likely to be the ward manager or a registered nurse. So good use of time is for the HCA to check against agreed stock numbers, consider what needs to be replaced and compose the order request. As the ward manager has trained the HCA in this task and has given her the responsibility to undertake it, signing the order form is a quick job. The ward manager has maintained accountability for supplies on the ward, but through effective delegation, training and devolved responsibility does not actually need to spend time looking over the store cupboards. The HCA is given responsibility which, as Maslow's hierarchy of needs (cited by Marquis and Huston, 2006) would indicate, is part of self-actualisation and a higher-level motivational factor and makes work more enjoyable.

Where there is over-delegation, the ward manager would have told the HCA to order the stock without training, support or monitoring and then wondered why problems subsequently arose or the HCA felt confused and stressed.

Improper delegation occurs when a manager asks a member of staff to undertake a task beyond his or her professional remit, for example, asking the HCA to sign the order form when she was not the budget-holder. Another example is the use of a student nurse to administer medication without trained staff supervision, which is also in disregard of the NMC *Code of Conduct* (2008b).

Assertiveness

Another area that should be considered alongside delegation is the concept of assertiveness, which is getting your point of view over without being aggressive. In the scenario when you asked the HCA to clean up the soiled patient, you were being assertive when you politely did not accept Ann's disinclination. Earlier in the chapter you will have used assertiveness, best illustrated by your body language, when you requested a discussion with the charge nurse concerning this and the HCAs' absence from the ward. Assertive communication is not aggression, which can be destructive, and might result in 'fight or flight' of those involved. On the contrary, it results in open dialogue and understanding while enhancing self-esteem. Nurses as a group have traditionally not been very assertive; they passively undertook tasks assigned to them, frequently by (often male) medical staff and did not voice their concerns. This passive role is no longer compatible with the nurse's role as an accountable practitioner (NMC, 2008b) but neither is an aggressive, domineering approach. The assertive nurse will politely but firmly communicate his or her wishes, feelings and thoughts to others but at the same time encourage dialogue. Assertiveness is a skill which can be learned. It is a behavioural technique, and should result in more self-confidence and better interpersonal relationships.

Conclusion

You can see that, as a newly qualified member of staff, you will be expected to act as a manager immediately and the way you demonstrate your leadership style will influence those around you. Being able to organise your workload, delegate activities and be assertive when required are all very important skills. You may have found it hard to undertake the second two in your student capacity.

The old adage 'you never get a second chance to make a first impression' applies in leadership situations as well as interviews.

Activities: brief outline answers

Activity 2.1

As a student you were encouraged to be accountable for your actions, but were always under the supervision of a trained nurse.

As a registered nurse you are accountable to the patient, your employer and your professional organisation.

Activity 2.2

It should be apparent that the main short-term problem is that, with the charge nurse and both experienced HCAs absent from the ward, both staff nurses will only have the ward clerk's knowledge of the unit in any emergency, which is not acceptable. It would have been much safer had the HCAs taken separate breaks, each accompanied by one of the staff nurses. This would have meant a trained nurse and an HCA, familiar with the ward routine, supported by the ward clerk would remain on the unit at all times. If the two staff nurses also decided to take their break together then the ward would be left unsafe, and if they went to break consecutively the morning breaks would be long overdue.

Activity 2.3

Remaining able to communicate in a professional manner can be very difficult when you feel that a situation is indicative of poor practice. You may have reflected that you would have felt unable to challenge the situation at all, particularly as the charge nurse doesn't seem to be taking you seriously. Alternatively you might have challenged the charge nurse straight away and been very assertive. In reality a more measured and planned approach is better.

Activity 2.4

Reasons for non-delegation include the following.

- It's quicker to do it myself.
- They might get it wrong.
- I don't have the confidence to ask someone else.
- They will feel that I am avoiding work.
- It means confronting other people.

Further reading and useful websites

humanresources.about.com/od/workrelationships/a/difficultpeople.htm

www.leadingpotential.com.au

www.managerialskills.org/management-tips-for-beginners/

www.methodcorp.com

These websites consider how to deal with difficult people at work and give ideas on how to manage at work.

www.scotland.gov.uk/Publications/2004/04/19299/36381

This is a helpful Scottish government paper on workload.

Chapter 3
Dealing with change

NMC Standards for Pre-registration Nursing Education

This chapter will address the following competencies:

Domain 2: Communication and interpersonal skills

4. All nurses must recognise when people are anxious or in distress and respond effectively, using therapeutic principles, to promote their wellbeing, manage personal safety and resolve conflict. They must use effective communication strategies and negotiation techniques to achieve best outcomes, respecting the dignity and human rights of all concerned. They must know when to consult a third party and how to make referrals for advocacy, mediation or arbitration.

Domain 4: Leadership, management and team working

All nurses must be professionally accountable and use clinical governance processes to maintain and improve nursing practice and standards of healthcare. They must be able to respond autonomously and confidently to planned and uncertain situations, managing themselves and others effectively. They must create and maximise opportunities to improve services. They must also demonstrate the potential to develop further management and leadership skills during their period of preceptorship and beyond.

NMC Essential Skills Clusters

This chapter will address the following ESCs:

Cluster: Organisational aspects of care

13. People can trust the newly registered graduate nurse to promote continuity when their care is transferred to another service or person.
18. People can trust a newly registered graduate nurse to enhance the safety of service users and identify and actively manage the risk and uncertainty in relation to people, the environment, self and others.
19. People can trust the newly registered graduate nurse to work to prevent and resolve conflict and maintain a safe environment.

Chapter aims

After reading this chapter, you will be able to:

* recognise the need for change in the workplace;
* discuss how change can be managed effectively;
* understand how individuals respond to change.

Introduction

Change is a very difficult concept to deal with in the workplace, although in reality our lives are full of change. The problems arise when we aren't the instigators of change but the passive recipients of something that happens to us. If we don't understand what is happening within the workplace or feel that our views are not being listened to, then we can become stressed.

Scenario

Towards the end of your nursing programme you were fortunate to be interviewed for a temporary post in the paediatric unit close to your home, but where your university did not have placements. At the interview it was stressed that your profile during the BSc Child Health programme had been exceptional and this was being taken into consideration, such that, despite being only newly qualified you were the chosen candidate. You were surprised, as other candidates seemingly had more experience but you had worked hard on your application form, portfolio and interview technique. Your student colleagues expressed their concerns that you wouldn't know the unit and that the post was only temporary, but you were clear that the advantages, paid work and a move home well exceeded any disadvantages, and you couldn't really believe your luck.

A fortnight before you are due to start this post, you get a letter from the paediatric unit manager Pat, asking you to meet with her as a matter of urgency; you are sure this will be bad news. You contact her secretary and are fortunate to be able to meet at the weekend, before you have a week's leave. Pat is very welcoming and starts to reassure you that this isn't bad news, but two changes are happening imminently and she wants to discuss these with you before you sign your contract.

Firstly Pat asks why you applied for a temporary post of only three months' duration; you explain that this would get you experience and an income, regardless of how short it was. She then asks if you would still consider this post if it was being made into a 12-month contract; you confirm your interest. Pat reminds you that the post was to cover a sabbatical experience for another junior nurse, who has now informed the unit that she is emigrating for good. Pat also adds that the human resources department (HR or personnel) has approved the change in length of the temporary post so that it doesn't need to be readvertised. You are delighted and are hard-pushed not to hug Pat, as the longer job security will be very helpful in dealing with your student debt.

Change in the workplace

Getting any first post is always difficult, but the importance of experience, no matter how little or different from the target, should always be seen as a positive step. Employers like to meet motivated, enthusiastic candidates who make use of their time and energy, even if it is not in the expected arena. By applying for a temporary post away from the area used for your training, you exhibit flexibility and adaptability, traits vital in effective workers. Had the post remained only very short-term, you would still have developed your trained nurse role and have more skills to offer to future employers. Even work that is unpaid or part-time will provide you with additional development and should never be discounted, even if it isn't ideal. The connections you make through any work may well reveal further opportunities or bring you to the notice of others.

It's not what you know but who you know may unfortunately apply as much today as it did in the early twentieth century.

Activity 3.1 — *Reflection*

Take the time to consider when you undertook an activity that had a surprising or useful outcome that you had not thought about when you started. Perhaps you started a new hobby that led to new friendships or skills that have influenced your life. Or perhaps a tutorial for a piece of academic work led to a clearer understanding of academic requirements and better marks thereafter.

As this is a personal reflection, no outline answer is supplied.

Scenario

Pat then says she wants to talk about the second change that will affect you once in post and you are rather mystified: now that you are being employed for a longer time, this can't be about the unit closing to save money. Pat talks about the need to reorganise the way services are delivered on the unit and to provide more care with an adolescent focus. You recall from your preapplication visit that the unit is a collection of small side wards, many of which are decorated to suit very young children, not the older ones; only the play leader seemed to be focused on the teenage patients.

Pat explains that she is telling you this before announcing it next week to the rest of the staff, as she is aware that it will not be a popular change and that as a new member of the team you would be 'walking in' on a proverbial hornet's nest. Pat asks that you don't discuss these changes with anyone else until she announces them.

As the meeting ends, you wonder what the rest of the team will think of the proposed change and whether they are at all aware of what is ahead.

Implementing change is difficult for any leader or manager and how this is carried out will affect how staff react to it and ultimately the success or failure of the proposals. In the scenario, the first change, extension of the temporary post, seems to be very minor and unlikely to cause problems. However Pat is wise to discuss this with you before you start the post: it may be that you had purposely taken a temporary post in order to fulfil other objectives, such as travel or further study, which would not be known to the employer. As Pat has already investigated any HR issues associated with changing the length of the temporary post contract, she is in a strong position when discussing this with you. It would have been a very different meeting if Pat needed to inform you that the post would be readvertised with details about its extension and that you would need to reapply.

With the approach that Pat is taking, she has justified your appointment to a longer-term post and made sure that this doesn't impinge on employment legislation or trust policy, before meeting you. She is making effective use of her time and her available resources, and will have a process to hand if you declined the change in employment. Importantly, you are also being consulted in this change; Pat is offering you alternatives, to accept or decline the offer, away from the workplace and before you feel under any obligation to accept. This is a well-managed change that Pat is able to pursue from her position of power.

Power is an interesting concept in the workplace: some power is expected, such as that of the unit manager. As a manager, Pat has power through a variety of roles: she is appointed to the post so she has legitimate power, and by the very nature of being the leader, she has power through connections to others ('who you know'). Pat has demonstrated her informational and expert power by seeking out processes and information prior to the meeting. Then, by demonstrating that she can offer you a change of contract that is to your benefit, she is illustrating power through reward; her friendly and approachable personality is likely to be admired by others and thus she achieves what is called referent power (La Monica, 1994).

Managing change

Scenario

You have been employed on the children's unit for two weeks before the day of the manager's scheduled meeting, when changes associated with the unit's reorganisation will be discussed. There has been a lot of speculation since the meeting was announced and you are aware that you are already party to some of the information. This has made you feel quite uncomfortable, as you weren't able to address some of the more outrageous concerns, such as closure of the unit or redundancies for staff.

Keeping organisational information secure or secret can sometimes be very difficult, as everyone likes to gossip. You will already be fully aware of the need for confidentiality concerning patient information, but may never have thought that organisations may also have secrets. You are grateful to Pat for having told you this information already, which demonstrates her trust in you. As she correctly surmised, you have yet to be integrated within the team and so would lack the peer support that is available to others.

The unit has a number of trained staff and some are very set in their ways. These are mainly the older staff, who delight in being 'sick children's nurses' and particularly in caring

continued . . .

for small babies. They have considerable expertise and enjoy sharing their knowledge wherever possible, yet they can see absolutely no point in having a specialist adolescent ward. Their belief seems to be that if children need to be treated for an 'adult illness', then they should be on an adult ward.

Pat is thus likely to face considerable disquiet when she describes the proposed changes. In order for the meeting to take place effectively, Pat has booked the day room and rearranged the furniture for the meeting. She has organised bank nursing staff to cover for the afternoon and the other paediatric senior manager from the community team within the trust will also be on the unit. In this way and by ensuring that all staff are on duty, Pat is able to inform the majority of staff in one sitting.

Activity 3.2   *Team working*

Have you ever been asked to attend a public or private meeting when you had no idea what the topic was about? How did you feel and what happened?

An outline answer is given at the end of the chapter.

Managing meetings

Setting up a meeting to get maximum attendance and thus involvement is a skill and Pat has rightly given thought to a lot of different aspects.

1. The venue needs to accommodate all the attendees reasonably and issues like room temperature, access to toilet facilities and IT resources should be considered.

2. The meeting must enable staff to be free to attend without interruption. Pat has booked staff from outside to cover the shift; with a local manager as an additional safeguard. Providing tea and biscuits, as this is an afternoon meeting, will add to the relaxed atmosphere, but should not be disruptive. Also, put a 'do not disturb' sign on the door and remind staff about silencing their mobile phones.

3. Unfortunately, it is never possible for everyone to attend a meeting, as some staff are likely to be off sick or on leave. The timing of any meeting should be such as to maximise potential attendance and the use of a note-taker or video recording will capture what has been said for those not present.

4. Taking notes or minutes from a meeting is really worthwhile, not just for those absent to catch up, but for those who attended to reflect on what was said. The notes should be made available promptly after the meeting, at least within the week, and should identify any actions needed, by whom and within what timeframe.

5. The difference between notes and minutes usually reflects the nature and regularity of the meeting. Typically, committee meetings will have minutes taken by a designated secretary, who will then write them up, check with the meeting chair and have them published. In contrast, an informal, one-off meeting may have a volunteer note-taker who captures the

essence of the meeting and then works with the meeting leader to write up the notes for distribution (Van Emden and Becker, 2004; Hall, 2007).

6. Getting the venue and 'housekeeping' issues correct from the start will help keep any meeting on track and may help boost the confidence of the meeting leader, as that person is demonstrating, at least to him- or herself, a level of control.

Scenario

Pat welcomes everyone to the meeting and asks that they sign the sheet, so that she can check on attendance and later for distribution of the minutes. She opens with recognising that just by calling the meeting she has caused alarm and distress and for that she apologises; she then explains that this is an important issue and everyone needs to understand the changes ahead.

Pat describes the situation at the moment which reflects complaints from families about the decor and style of much of the unit, as it is too baby-focused. She explains that caring for sick adolescent children has been a growth area for which there needs to be specialist equipment and resources. She also shows statistics on bed occupancy of the cots, for children under one year old, in light of the development of the regional special care baby unit in a nearby trust.

Pat then asks for questions and comments from the audience and the first ones reflect job insecurities – 'Will the unit be closing then?' and 'Are we being made redundant?' Pat clearly reiterates that there are changes planned, but that closure and redundancy are not the objectives. There is a good deal of muttering and some non-verbal communication which suggest a lack of belief in what has been said, but Pat allows this to continue for a few minutes, whilst the staff internalise what they have heard.

Pat is effectively managing the meeting because she is aware that unless the staff are given the opportunity to voice their feelings, it will be impossible to get her message across. Pat then addresses any specific questions that reflect reasonable concerns, before informing the group that she wants to move the meeting forward. During the discussion one of the administrative staff has taken down notes summarising the main concerns.

As the manager, Pat is fully aware of the trust's plans for the unit and recognises that she is acting as the go-between in what could be a difficult situation. So she starts by reiterating what overall changes are planned and then asks for suggestions as to how this could take place. In particular, she asks for suggestions on the unit layout, which aspects work currently and which do not. In this way, although the number of small rooms with cots will alter anyway, other layout improvements could occur concurrently.

Activity 3.3   *Critical thinking*

Think back to a situation in your own life – it may well be outside work – where you were forced to change. For instance, your parents moved house and you had to change schools or you moved home and work with your partner's job. How did you feel: were you angry or frustrated?

An outline answer is provided at the end of the chapter.

Managing change can be very difficult because, as Lewin points out in his seminal work, individuals always resist change, perceiving that the status quo is a safer place than the unknown. Change is disruptive at a whole range of levels and, as Maslow's hierarchy of motivational needs reflects, concerns about employment are about meeting the lowest level of physical and safety needs and these are the foundation level (Figure 3.1) (Lewin and Maslow, cited by Marquis and Huston, 2006).

Thus, if staff are reassured that they are still employed after a change, they may be more open to considering the issues; however, the hierarchy of needs clearly applies at other levels beyond physical and security needs, which are also linked to work. Working patterns provide staff with social networks and affiliations, colleagues with whom they not only spend time at work but may have as friends outside. Similarly and importantly in this scenario, their self-esteem and self-worth (self-actualisation) may be closely linked with their expertise in baby care. Experienced staff, who have a good reputation in the arena of baby care, may feel very concerned about their inability to deal with adolescents, their illnesses and social needs. It is thus important that even if a change doesn't result in unemployment, which is currently a real concern, it may still undermine feelings of self-worth and self-esteem and so is resisted.

Lewin also considered what drove change and what caused people to resist change: he termed this a force-field analysis. He explained that change would only occur if the driving forces

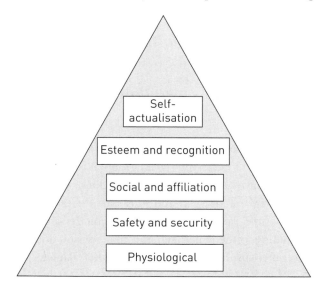

Figure 3.1. Maslow's hierarchy of needs. The lowest-level needs have to be met first. Issues associated with employment affect staff at many levels: at the lowest level, it provides a wage to buy food and other essentials.

exceeded the resisting forces and, importantly for managers, it is reducing the resisting forces that is critical to success. Unfortunately, many managers see that they should only enhance the driving forces and that this will eventually overcome any resistance, rather than trying to reduce the resistance.

This can be well illustrated by considering a war situation such as the so-called Arab spring uprisings of 2011. Even though the individual official governments have the fire power to overcome the opposition armies, they are not able to destroy the opposition completely. The resistance, underground or terrorist faction, continues to fight, until the government accepts the situation and agrees to a change through compromise and a cease-fire is reached.

Each manager in any situation needs to identify the driving and resisting forces and Pat will have thought about this before her meeting. By holding a meeting that all can attend, Pat has ensured that the same message is being heard by everyone and this should help to reduce some of the more outrageous or imagined concerns that arise from individuals.

Hersey and Blanchard, in La Monica (1994), describe how there are levels of change which are progressively more difficult to manage; it is more difficult to guarantee a planned outcome the more people who are involved and over a longer period of time.

In considering the change levels, Pat will recognise that updating staff in their knowledge of the care needed by adolescents and their families is a fairly routine task that may involve some teaching sessions by experts and some self-studying. However, the attitude and behaviour of individuals are likely to be linked to Maslow's higher motivational needs, such as loss of self-esteem and self-worth. Staff will feel that all their years of experience are being undervalued and that perhaps this is a way of getting them to leave the organisation. Clearly, once individuals communicate their concerns to each other, the staff will illustrate group behaviour, which is unhelpful but self-perpetuating and frequently destructive. Pat needs the staff to participate in the proposed changes at the lowest levels in the first instance, and that is at the knowledge level, which is why she has started by explaining what is proposed rather than what is imagined.

Other researchers on change also consider how change is resisted if it is imposed top-down rather than grown from the bottom up. To this end Pat needs to involve the staff in what is happening and maximise their feelings of ownership of the change, which is why she has asked for people's ideas on the unit design.

Scenario

Pat supplies some sticky notes and flip chart paper to capture ideas and asks staff to be creative, regardless of how artistic they are. You start to lead your small group: it is still not apparent to the others that this is not the first you have heard of the proposals. This exercise aims to allow a freedom of ideas and to get everyone involved and thus start the task of ownership of the change – the start of a bottom-up approach. Pat sits quietly while everyone works alone or in small groups, listening to the general chatter that goes on and fully aware that some staff see this activity as time-wasting. After about 15 minutes, Pat asks

continued . . .

everyone to give feedback on what they have drawn or listed and explain their thoughts so that there can be an effective group discussion before closure. Pat wants the meeting to close on time, as staff will have other commitments to attend to and a late finish may elicit bad feeling, and she needs the meeting to end on a positive note. She thanks everyone and gathers their paper work up to look at in more detail, and reminds the staff that she wants to hear their views further and for them to feel free to contact her.

Pat takes the participants' notes home, along with the administrators' jottings, and starts to put the ideas into useful areas which will also create the meeting feedback to her staff and her own manager. As you leave the meeting, Pat asks if you have a few minutes to spare to discuss your progress on the unit.

As a manager it is important to support new members of staff in any situation and Pat will have been aware that you have had to keep the information you knew confidential, which will have been challenging. Organisations frequently need members of staff to keep 'secrets' and this can result in a stressful situation for all concerned, so as a manager it is important to provide a debrief on a situation that may have caused undue stress. She is aware that you will have had more time to consider the issue and it will have been difficult not to talk about the changes when others will have been making wild suppositions. In the scenario Pat has attempted to get everyone involved in the idea of change; this will not be an easy step to take and some staff will fail to see the value of the meeting. Your views on the event will be useful to her and also offer an opportunity for her to praise you on maintaining confidentiality and ask about your general progress on the unit.

Managers should always be aware that individuals accept change at different rates and that this will need to be dealt with effectively if the whole team is to be supported and guided through the changes. The implementer of any change, frequently but not always the manager, needs to get those in the organisation to accept the change and implement it. Lewin identifies that the move to implementation is not straightforward and has three phases.

The first stage is to *unfreeze* existing practice; this invariably means getting the staff or team to think about the problem and consider changing practice. Unfreezing is more difficult than many implementers believe and the use of information, displays and talks may enable this to happen, but frequently a more long-term and persistent approach is needed, getting the idea into the group's psyche. In the scenario, Pat has undertaken part of the unfreezing phase by getting all the staff together and talking to them and asking for their views; she is thus providing external motivation towards her goals. She will now need to work with all the individual members of staff to address their concerns and encourage them to have internal motivation towards the goals. The move from external to internal motivation will parallel a move from top-down to bottom-up change implementation.

The next stage is the *change* phase, when staff are *primed to accept the new patterns of behaviour* (La Monica, 1994, p193) and, in the presence of the implementer, will undertake the new ways of working or behaving. The members of staff will practise the new ways of working and are seen to be internalising the change.

Refreezing only occurs when the new ways of working are so integrated that they take place instinctively and without any external motivators being present. The change is now integral to the way the team works routinely (Figure 3.2).

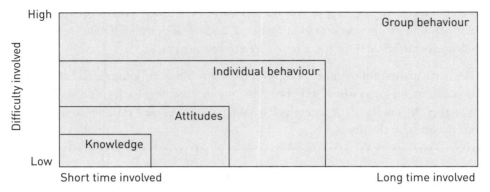

Figure 3.2. The process of change (adapted from Lewin's model), showing how the most difficult changes involve the most people over the longest time.

Activity 3.4   *Communication*

Consider a situation where change has been implemented. Was this done successfully?

An outline answer is provided at the end of the chapter.

How people deal with change

Staff accept change at different rates. Much of the work in this area came from marketing theory, and may be understood more easily when related to items such as mobile phones or the iPad or iPod. However, it can also be applied to the dynamics of change adoption in the workplace.

Those most willing to change are the *innovators*: they are enthusiastic and thrive on any change, although they may well become easily bored and move on to the next new thing. The innovator may well have been queuing at his local Apple store at midnight, for the first-generation iPad to be released!

Next are the *early adopters*. These are individuals who will embrace change easily and often enjoy the challenges of new things but would wait to hear the first reviews on the iPad before buying it. An exploration of these early adopters will probably reveal that their attitude to work change is mirrored in their social situation; they like new challenges and new technology and tend to have 'cutting-edge' equipment. These two groups of staff will really assist the implementer.

Late adopters are those individuals who will give rather more consideration to any change before accepting it. These people are more likely to wait for critical reviews of new gadgets or the second release (the iPad 2) before purchasing something new, to see what difficulties have now been resolved.

The *early and late majority* are those who will wait until a change is fairly firmly established and, where goods are concerned, the price has fallen considerably before they accept the change or make the purchase. They take a variable time to be convinced but once they accept the change will be strongly committed and maintain the change.

Those who are more difficult to work with are the *laggards*. These are unlikely to change without some further incentive. In the mobile phone industry, for instance, these individuals will have been given a phone for emergencies or provided with one free, but will make minimal use now they own it.

The *rejecters* are the most difficult group to manage in marketing. They are the small percentage that won't ever make the purchase and may actually campaign against something.

In the workplace laggards may need continual reminders to change practice, particularly if the implementer or supervisor is absent; otherwise they revert to old behaviour. The rejecters are the most difficult group to manage in the workplace as they can be terribly disruptive, and may set out to sabotage any proposed or implemented change. Sometimes they will have genuine concerns about a change, but often it is more intangible and reflects a reliance on past ways of working. Historically, the Luddites who smashed mechanised looms fitted into this category; they couldn't stop progress but did what they could to obstruct it (Bushy and Kamphuis, 1993, in Marquis and Huston, 1994, p179).

Activity 3.5   *Decision-making*

Are you an early adopter or a laggard? Think about the way you or your family members respond to new gadgets on the high street. Do you function the same way with organisational change?

An outline answer is provided at the end of the chapter.

How individuals accept change will affect the success of any proposal and, as the implementer, it is vital to recognise these different rates of adoption. Early adopters are enthusiastic and keen for change and thus in the first stages will be dynamic and willing, but they do get bored easily and move to a new challenge. Laggards may need to be carefully monitored for some considerable time after the implementation of the change, as they may not have embedded changes and failed to move to the refreeze phase. Rejecters are even more difficult and, if they continue to cause major disruption and distress to the rest of the team, they may need to face disciplinary action or move to another work setting where they fit in better.

Kotter and Schlesinger (1979, cited by McSherry and Pearce, 2002, p 101) described four main reasons why individuals resist change:

1. parochial self-interest: they might lose something of value;
2. misunderstanding or lack of trust: they might lose more than they gain by any change;
3. different assessments: they see costs more than benefits for the whole organisation;
4. low tolerance for change: they fear not having the correct skills or behaviour.

In the scenario Pat will have some members of the team who are likely to be willing to accept the change in working practice and she may feel that as you are newly qualified this will apply to you. There will be others for whom the change is unwanted and resisted on many levels and for whom the external motivation will not override the internal (de)motivation.

Pat's next task is to consider what the meeting and the feedback have told her in terms of good ideas and staff motivation. If Pat can use ideas put forward by her staff, then she will be using a bottom-up approach and this is more likely to have a positive outcome.

Scenario

One of the suggestions written on a sticky note is for statistics on the incidence of babies and adolescents on the unit and thus the need for the change. Pat recognises that this is really useful information that she hasn't publicised, even though it is the driving top-down force from the trust, so she immediately gets these figures made available to staff. A graph showing the dramatic shift in the type of clients since the opening of the special care baby unit is very clear and makes a strong point for a reduction in cots, which are placed in separate small cubicles. The continued increase in teenage occupancy, although less dramatic in the short term, is very marked over the last three years.

Another staff comment is the lack of understanding on the social and play needs of today's teenagers, as some of the staff either have grown-up children or are not yet parents. Pat decides to set up a talk by some of those who are particularly knowledgeable in teenage care and invite one of the 'expert' adolescent patients to meet the staff, and she will record the meeting so that everyone can view it, even if not on duty.

The trust has estimated that the building work will happen over a four-week period and the team agree that this should be in the summer holidays. At this time staffing can always be difficult, due to annual leave requests from the nurses. There are also fewer medical admissions and the day theatre cleaning closure can be planned to coincide. This recommendation is taken forward, as it also allows for some flexibility and over-run and is being suggested by the workforce.

After the 'teenage' training session has taken place, a few more staff indicate that the changes proposed might actually be good for the unit and that they will appreciate the redecoration and updating of the building.

Pat reconsiders her force-field analysis of the change. There now appear to be far fewer restraining forces and the drivers have been strengthened. She also gives thought to her process of change (Figure 3.2); she recognises that the knowledge and attitudes of many staff have moved considerably and that some individual behaviour shows commitment to the new ways of working. However, she is aware that individuals may not be as open about their commitment as she has hoped and that until the changes are in place, the group behaviour may still be unpredictable or even destructive.

Bennis et al. (1969, cited by Marquis and Huston, 2006) consider that the change agent (Pat in the scenario) can use a variety of change strategies to influence behaviour. These are rational–empirical, normative–re-educative and power–coercive.

When managers support a *rational–empirical* strategy, they believe that providing the facts and documentation will automatically persuade the workers to change, as they too will behave rationally. In the scenario the provision of bed usage and occupancy charts supports this process and it will influence some staff.

Using the *normative–re-educative* strategy means recognising that peer pressure and social norms and routines need to be influenced or altered in order to make change. Pat brings in expert staff to talk about the difference in working practices; she develops the confidence of her staff and doesn't make them feel undervalued.

Finally, the *power–coercive* strategy relies on rewards and punishments; managers using this technique believe that staff have to be forced into a change. Pat will be alert to the knowledge that the trust will make the changes, whether the staff like it or not, and that ultimately she may have to move staff who refuse to care for adolescents, but it is not the method she wants to use.

Thus in reality Pat, like many managers, will use a variety of strategies to influence the way staff feel about changes, so that these changes can be implemented in a painfree way.

Pat will hope that the meeting and feedback will have helped reduce McSherry and Pearce's (2002) four resistances, by providing better understanding of the process and planning involved, but she still cannot guarantee the outcome. Unfortunately, as change occurs in all aspects of private and working life, the leader or change implementer needs to use the various strategies to make this happen effectively. The healthcare systems of today are in constant flux, with multiple small changes for which the outcomes cannot always be predicted.

The unpredictable nature of change in organisations has been named chaos theory; this was a term coined by Edward Lorenz in 1960 with regard to the weather (cited by Bach and Ellis 2011). Lorenz noted that a rise in sea temperature in one area altered the airflow and thus the winds in another area, something which could not have been predicted – chaos. The manager's role is thus to look at all aspects of a proposed change and to try to manage them and limit harmful outcomes, while recognising that there will be unexpected results.

The workers on the 'shop floor' frequently know far better than those in management how well existing systems work and where they are flawed and so will have good ideas about potential improvements. The ideas from the 'shop floor' must be considered realistically by managers as they are frequently based on sound judgment and the resultant changes will have an element of the bottom-up approach.

In the scenario Pat has introduced the concept of the planned change. By repeated meetings, posters and involving the staff in small decisions she should get them to 'own' the change. Typically, getting staff to consider the room layouts, colour schemes and timing of the change implementation is important; because this engenders ownership of the change, which will be needed if the change is to be implemented successfully. Once this major change has been implemented, Pat can show how the staff have participated at various stages and influenced the changes, albeit in small ways. The ability of an organisation to adapt to small and frequent changes, as a series of small steps, is a very constructive and an effective way to work. This is likely to lead to greater success and happier staff, who respond positively to future change.

Activities: brief outline answers

Activity 3.2

It is likely that you were anxious about the outcome, particularly if the meeting was important for yourself, your family or work. You might also have been aware that there was considerable gossip or speculation in the press about what the meeting might mean.

With hindsight you might consider that you could have been better prepared for the meeting, by doing some reading or online searches.

If you were surprised by the meeting's content, did you make notes to follow up later? Were you able to ask the question for which you needed clarity?

Activity 3.3

Although this is in part a reflection, it is really asking you to be critical of your own reactions to change. As a child you may have felt that moving house would mean loss of friends and social life, particularly if this was before the advent of electronic networking tools! As an adult, moving with one's partner's job can seem reasonable if it provides job security or more income, but it can also cause disruption and upset – loss of friends and networks.

Activity 3.4

Did you consider a clinical workplace situation where change had been successfully introduced? One change that has been successfully implemented in many areas is 'bare below the elbows' to reduce cross-infection and encourage hand-washing. This change has involved both top-down governmental directives on reducing cross-infection and a bottom-up approach that involves all staff, regardless of grade.

Activity 3.5

So what did you decide about your own responses to change? Did you recognise yourself as at either extreme end of the change adoption spectrum, as an innovator or a rejecter or somewhere in between? This will affect the way you interact at work or home, when changes occur or are requested. You may believe that you are being logical when you respond to changes in a particular way, but please give it some thought.

Further reading and useful websites

Baulcomb, JS (2003) Management of change through force field analysis. **www.fchs.ac.ae/fchs/uploads/Files/Semester%201%20-%202010-2011/4120/Change_Force_Field_Analysis.pdf**.

Lorch, A (2007) Implementation of fasting guidelines through nursing leadership. **www.nursingtimes.net/nursing-practice-clinical-research/implementation-of-fasting-guidelines-through-nursing-leadership/201890.article**.

www.nwlink.com/~donclark/leader/leadcon.html

Big Dog and Little Dog's performance juxtaposition website on management and leadership.

www.businessballs.com/changemanagement.htm

This is a helpful source for change management theory.

Chapter 4
Working with staff: your role as a leader

> **Chapter aims**
>
> After reading this chapter, you will be able to:
>
> - recognise situations where leadership is required;
> - demonstrate leadership traits yourself.

Introduction

In this chapter you will learn about some of the theories that have developed around leadership and how they are believed to influence the way staff within organisations function. All organisations have managers who run them and some of these managers are also leaders, directing the staff towards goals which fit with the company objectives.

Leadership and management

Healthcare is an organisation made up of a great many disparate parts and needs to be managed and led at all levels of the hierarchy. For instance, you might believe that healthcare has only one objective, making people better, so that all employees would be striving towards this goal, but in reality healthcare could be about treating illness or perhaps it should be primarily about preventing disease. If you are the charge nurse in a busy accident and emergency department, trying to treat a road traffic accident victim, you will have very different objectives to those of a health visitor checking babies for normal development. The leader in either clinical situation will demonstrate different priorities and help the team meet its objectives as effectively as possible. Leadership happens at all levels within an organisation and leaders are not always in positions of power or prestige, but they do have objectives. For instance, the nursing auxiliary, who is also the trade union shop steward, may well exhibit with her colleagues power and influence more commensurate with that of a nurse manager.

Organisations rely on their staff to work to the best of their abilities to achieve the organisational goals and it is the leaders and managers who help direct this. Management and leadership have elements that overlap; some authors suggest that leadership is about people while management is about tasks. Clearly, the two are interrelated and good leadership can be found in a good manager and vice versa.

> **Scenario**
>
> Since you completed your student nursing programme as a mature student, you have made the decision to work locally rather than travel to the district general hospital, where you did much of your training. Some of your fellow students feel that it is vital to get a post in a dynamic unit or busy ward to gain specialist skills, but you are not sure they are right. You

continued . . .

have recognised the need to consolidate and build on your existing skills and also that your family might appreciate you being at home a bit more.

You recently responded to an advertisement in the local paper and were subsequently appointed as a staff nurse at a local nursing home; this was your first choice of work and you are really pleased. You enjoy caring for older people as they have complex nursing needs, but you have also found working with their families, general practitioners and other social care organisations rewarding. Sometimes you wonder whether your colleagues actually have as much day-to-day responsibility as you do, in their high-tech intensive care unit posts – you somehow doubt it.

The home has recently changed owners and is now registered as a nursing home rather than residential care. These terms have recently changed: the Care Quality Commission (CQC) recognises former nursing homes as 'care homes with nursing', i.e. providing personal care, medication and nursing care and with a registered nurse available 24 hours a day (**www.guidanceaboutcompliance.org.uk/step1.php**). A residential care home is now known as simply as a care home. You are among a number of relatively new appointees and one of the most recently qualified, also the only graduate, but many of your colleagues don't know this, as your age and past experiences suggest otherwise.

Activity 4.1   *Team working*

Were you typical of the students in your cohort? Did you fit in well or find that your background, age or life experiences singled you out? Consider how this affected your relationships with your peers, tutors or practice areas.

Do you categorise people by their appearance?

It is important that you consider how others see you, as this may affect your perceived leadership style or how colleagues treat you.

As this is a personal reflection, no outline answer is given.

Types of leadership

Can you always tell who is naturally a leader?

Throughout history, people have required leaders to help direct group activities towards a shared goal; in prehistoric times it might have been the strongest caveman who led the tribe, because of his physical abilities. Writers in history sometimes comment that certain individuals born into powerful dynasties were destined to be leaders; their ability to lead was a birthright. These leaders ruled their empires, because they were great men (or sometimes great women); they were believed to know instinctively the right course of action. History has demonstrated that this can clearly be untrue and modern writers on leadership disregard this concept.

Weber in 1947 (cited by Marquis and Huston, 2006) wrote about the *rational* base for leadership, describing how the social norm supports the power base, for example, a belief in the monarchy as natural leaders. Weber also described a *traditional* base, where leadership and power have always come from a particular source, such as the landed gentry or the church, and the mass population believes this is as it should be. Popular culture would add 'older equals wiser' to indicate that leadership comes with age and experience in any social situation, but again this is clearly not true. Weber's final view was that there was are *charismatic leaders*, heroes or heroines, who know the right thing to do and thus 'weaker' individuals will instinctively follow them in times of trouble.

Other slightly more recent writers believed that it was an individual's *charismatic personality* that produced leadership skills through great oration. Unfortunately, although these personality traits may inspire others, it may not always be to the good. Personality does affect leadership, as being able to voice your objection to those in power is a useful tool, but it is not of primary importance.

Not all historical perspectives should be discarded automatically. Machiavelli wrote his treatise *The Prince* about power and influence in fifteenth-century Italy, and this text has as much relevance today as it did then. He wrote about power and leadership as the flow of information between the warring nobility. In modern terms 'machiavellian' suggests cunning and underhand behaviour, but in fact Machiavelli wrote about ways of behaving and leading with those who were friends or enemies. He recognised that the use of effective communication is paramount to good leadership.

Reading an English translation of Machiavelli's work is surprisingly easy, and, more intriguingly, clearly relevant today!

In the scenario, there may be a misconception that you, being a mature entrant to the profession, are 'older and wiser' and thus a natural leader based on your experience. This might be coupled with the *rational* view, as you have a degree as well as registration and thus leadership attributes. However, more recent writers would suggest that good leaders 'rise to the occasion'; they reflect the needs of the task in hand and as such are the *situational leader*. This hypothesis would identify a different leader appropriate for each different situation, but that doesn't necessarily happen and in reality it is likely that leaders have a combination of all the traits.

Consider, for instance, a girl who is born into royalty; there may be an expectation that she is a natural leader – as she has wealth and power leadership will be inherent – but this isn't the case. What does occur is that she is given the best education money can buy, which instils leadership through activities such as becoming school prefect, sports captain or head girl. These roles further develop confidence and power, already 'inherited' from birth, and which are then demonstrated in the girl's life experiences. In reality, it wasn't that the individual inherited leadership skills through her genes, but that expectation and opportunity developed them. Clearly not all leaders have this type of upbringing and education: some are the direct opposite, the 'street urchin' determined by sheer willpower to become a success against all the odds. In the world of work, it may be that leadership comes from unexpected directions.

Recognising situations needing leadership

Scenario

You have been working at the home for several weeks now and have started to feel that there are areas of nursing care that really need to be changed. It is not that care has been particularly poor, but staff don't work in a systematic or logical way, to the extent that clients may not be ready to go to the dining room at lunch time. Colleagues who started work at the home at much the same time as you also express concern at the way some of the established staff work. There is Nicky, a young woman who moved to this area with her fiancé and his job, who expects to be looking for a post in the district general hospital once she has established a home. Patience is an experienced Filipino nurse, who has returned to full-time work now that both her children have started school, and you are the oldest of the three, but actually least experienced professionally.

You are all fully aware that this is the clients' home, so routines should be flexible to accommodate client requests, but this is not at the root of the problem, which is having a detrimental effect on patient care. Nicky also asks what you think about the drug administration system and you have to confess that you've given it less thought, but do recognise the potential for problems. Patience feels that you should not challenge the situation, as you are all new to post and jobs are hard to find; she is concerned you might lose yours by 'making trouble'. You and Nicky reassure Patience that not only do you all have obligations professionally (NMC, 2008b) to look at the standards of care, but employment law in the UK should protect you.

You agree to ask for a meeting with Kim, the newly appointed home manager, who is not a nurse, to discuss your concerns and consider a way forward.

Activity 4.2   *Decision-making*

What would you do if you observed working practices that were not as good as they could be, or at risk of causing harm? You have an obligation under law to follow this up.

An outline answer is provided at the end of the chapter.

You and Nicky recognise that the nursing care situation needs to be challenged and changed; there has been too little leadership. Kim recognises that she needs a situational leader and one who is a clinical nurse, even though as home manager she would be the traditional or rational leader, as she has power and status. What Kim lacks in this situation is the knowledge and expertise to communicate nursing issues with the team, some of whom will welcome the changes (Machiavelli's 'friends') and some who will contest it ('enemies').

In the scenario, two concepts should come to mind concerning management: the first is the need to *change* established practice; the second is that you are already showing strands of leadership. You are not the leader by birthright or by being an *authoritative figure*. As a newly appointed staff member the social order would not indicate you as the natural leader so the rational/traditional view does not apply and you may or may not be charismatic! So the leadership that you are demonstrating in the scenario is one arising from the situation, which you feel empowered to change; but also with Nicky you illustrate a *collaborative* process.

Girvin (1998) summarises the leadership theories as based on four areas:

1. innate personal qualities;
2. specific behaviour and activities;
3. contingency or contextual response to a situation;
4. group/relationship, a collaborative and interactive process.

The fourth theme is how the leadership, by two staff nurses, is developing in the scenario. Recalling Chapter 3, on change, you should recall that as you are actually working with the client group (the 'product') on the 'shop floor', your changes are being proposed in a bottom-up way.

Demonstrating leadership traits

Scenario

Kim readily agrees to a meeting the following afternoon, in her office; Patience offers to remain with the clients so that you and Nicky aren't disturbed. You wonder if this is really altruistic behaviour on her part or concerns about her employment; however, you thank her for being so helpful. In the meeting Kim asks you both how you have settled in and then goes on to apologise for having spent so little time together. Kim describes her background and admits that she has had to leave all the nursing care to her staff, while she considered all the other issues associated with running the home, since she has only been in post a fortnight longer than you. Kim says her background is in hotel work and not nursing; she also explains that within reasonable financial boundaries she is more than happy to delegate to the nursing staff. Kim says she had been given the power, in financial terms, to increase the capacity of the home but that to do this requires an effective team. She too has noticed the chaotic nature of some mornings, when the doorbell seems to ring non-stop and clients have had to eat lunch in their rooms. She asks you both what you want to do.

In the scenario, it is apparent that the home manager is the figure of authority and should thus be the leader, but it is also clear that in terms of nursing practice Kim accepts that she is neither the manager nor the leader: that role falls to you or Nicky.

Adair, writing in 1988 (cited by Girvin, 1998), explained that power in organisations comes from the position held, the knowledge held or the personality of the individual. So considering the scenario, Kim as the home manager should hold *positional power* as it comes from one's place in the hierarchy of an organisation. The higher up the hierarchy the 'boss' is, the greater her authority and decision-making capacity. Kim is a wise manager: she may recognise that she has the ultimate organisational responsibility and accountability, but she isn't a nurse and thus doesn't undertake nursing.

You and Nicky on the other hand have *knowledge power*, which comes from your nursing registration and practice credibility. You are thus managers who understand the issues of the business (nursing), and can provide leadership through expertise, despite not being the boss.

Any or all of you – Nicky, Kim and yourself – may have *personality power* and *charisma*, and can influence the staff, though this is often seen as exuberance, enthusiasm and charm. Thus individuals who can attract attention and good will, at least in the short term, have leadership. However, there does also need to be positional or knowledge-based power to support this; power in all three arenas will make a very effective leader. As an effective manager, Kim will demonstrate some abilities in all three areas: she has positional power as home manager; knowledge power, from her experience in hotels; and personality power through her positive attitude to the senior nursing staff. As Kim freely recognises the limits of her knowledge and lack of nursing expertise and asks your opinion, she is making a conscious effort to empower the qualified staff. As staff nurses in a nursing home, most of those undertaking nursing tasks will be auxiliaries or healthcare assistants; these people need leadership and it is the staff nurses who must supply it.

However, Kelemen (2003) makes the important link that no matter how you classify leadership styles or approaches, the effect on the quality of healthcare (or 'products manufactured') is what ultimately matters most to an organisation. Kim in the scenario is recognising that her senior nursing staff have the ability and responsibility to change nursing practice. As staff nurses in this situation you will demonstrate leadership and hence manage the nursing care.

Scenario

As you and Nicky leave the meeting with Kim, you realise that what she has done is to leave the changes and the leadership of the nursing team with you. It is going to be up to you two, hopefully with the support of Patience, to lead the nursing care forward. Patience states that she is quite happy to follow any direction you and Nicky suggest, but doesn't want to make the decisions as she finds this too stressful. You and Nicky think that the next step will be to sit down and 'brainstorm' what the problems are and so agree to meet after work one evening.

When you meet up, there seem so many issues that neither of you knows quite where to start, so you discuss the issues associated with change management and small stepwise changes rather than big leaps to get everyone on board. You also discuss how the other staff are going to behave when you try to make changes and where the problems may lie. Nicky expresses her concern that, as she is only in her early twenties and straight from university, she won't appear to have the gravitas to be taken seriously. She is surprised when you admit that you were a mature entrant to nursing and also haven't been registered very long, but that this was your preferred type of employment.

continued . . .

After you have written lots of notes about what you both perceive as problems, you construct a 'wish list' in priority order. The first is the safety of the patients with their medication; the second the scheduling of each morning's work. You both believe that Kim will accept your recommendations for safer medicines management, provided you undertake a *cost–benefit analysis*. You both know that the *costs* to Kim and the home-owners of buying new drug storage systems need to balance against the *benefits* of safe practice and a reduction in drug errors. Nicky says that she will take the lead in this problem as she is happy to research drug storage and supply systems. You both know that Patience and the other trained staff, who work part-time day or night duty, will be happy with whatever you decide about medication, and that Kim will be convinced by the cost–benefit findings.

Cost–benefit analysis in management

A cost–benefit analysis is a way to work out the positives and negatives of any change, and should include all manner of issues, not just financial ones. A good leader must be able to explain the rationale for action, to demonstrate that it is not based on a whim. In this cost–benefit analysis it is apparent that there are benefits to both systems, but the overall objective is to recognise and tackle 'costs' – the actual problems – rather than just forgetting them in the enthusiasm for the change.

For instance, as Nicky is making the recommendation about changing the drug dispensing system from generic boxes and bottles to patient-specific bubble pack, she presents the following cost–benefit analysis. This considers the advantages in terms of money, staff time and patient safety of the two systems and Nicky argues that the final two benefits have to be seen long-term and as potential major financial savings (Table 4.1).

Managing change in teams

Scenario

At your planned evening meeting, you and Nicky discuss how you will lead the changes. You are both concerned that the most risks to the clients, and thus ultimately the home itself, come from the medicines management problems. You decide together that you will need to take an authoritarian approach to leading in a situation where safe practice must be maintained. You are both aware that this authoritarian model of leadership (as suggested by Lewin in the early 1960s: **www.encyclopedia.com/topic/Kurt_Lewin.aspx**) is not popular and doesn't lead to self-motivation. Yet without some enforced changes to practice, care is going to be compromised. Nicky rapidly investigates the cost of a new drug storage system and asks the local pharmacist to visit the home. It is also to become policy that only registered nurses administer drugs, even though the assistants had done this in the residential home. You both recognise that this isn't going to be popular with some of the experienced carers who will feel demoted and resent this loss of status.

Costs and benefits of old drug administration system	Costs and benefits of new drug administration system
Generic supplies mean that there may be too much of a medicine to use in a reasonable time period	Specific bubble pack for each individual patient reduces waste
Old-style storage provided generic stock for emergencies	May need to provide small emergency stock – negative financial implication
Contamination of supplies is a problem	No contamination between patients with bubble packs and decreased risk of cross-infection
Staff are familiar with the old storage system, but this will need replacing eventually	Need to purchase specific drug storage system for bubble packs – negative financial implication
No way of checking accurate usage levels, potential for theft of supplies	Bubble packs permit easy checking of numbers of pills administered
Any pharmacy usable	Need arrangement with local pharmacy to supply bubble packs which may have financial implications but may improve working relationship with specific pharmacy
Generic drug containers are cheaper to supply	Bubble packs may be costly
High risk of drug errors relating to dosage and individual prescription	Reduced risk of drug errors with bubble packs
Difficult to prove drugs have been administered correctly	Reduced risk of complaints about drug maladministration

Table 4.1. Cost–benefit analysis of change to drug system in the nursing home

It should be seen that in this comparison (Table 4.1) the most important driving forces are the actual costs of the new storage systems versus the potential costs of drug administration errors. From a professional point of view and with concerns about patient safety, the drug administration system should override issues of cost, but a good case may need to be made to the management.

What drug administration and storage methods have you seen? How does each method ensure the safe administration of medication? Are some better in this regard than others?

An outline answer is provided at the end of the chapter.

Scenario

As you and Nicky must lead the nursing care changes, it is clear that the rest of the staff must be convinced that they are in everyone's best interest; this requires leadership. When Nicky brings in a new drug administration and storage system, she can utilise an authoritarian leadership style, with the support and power of the home manager. This change has to be made as client safety is paramount and there can be little negotiation or discussion. Nicky has used her knowledge to rationalise the proposed change to Kim and the nursing home owners; she can use a normative–educative approach to implement the changes.

Some managers believe that workers needed to be controlled; that they need to be coerced into doing what the manager wants; that staff need direction, lack motivation and need to be told what to do at all times. McGregor, writing in 1960 (cited by Marquis and Huston, 2006), proposed this theory X model, where all the power rests with the leader who directs and controls the workers. This has some relevance today, in some emergency situations, as it can be vital that all staff must follow a unified procedure very quickly. However, the view that staff are immature and not self-motivating has been dismissed, as illustrated by the way you and Nicky, in the scenario, have recognised a need to lead and change working practices.

Theory summary: theory X and Y

Theory Y-style managers believe that employees are self-motivated, they find work and new experiences challenging and are creative and self-controlling. Clearly the kind of leadership required if staff behave according to theory Y is very different from theory X.

McGregor summarised that the personality traits affecting theory X and theory Y behaviour in the workplace (**www.businessballs.com/mcgregor.htm**), and thus the leadership needed, are:

- work attitude;
- ambition;
- creativity;
- motivation;
- control.

Individuals exhibited various degrees of these traits.

A similar view of how individuals behave in an organisation and thus the way they need to be led is found in Argyris' (1971, cited by La Monica, 1994) immaturity–maturity continuum. This theory also considered personality traits at work:

- work attitude;
- dependence;
- behaviour;
- interests;
- concern;
- position;
- self-awareness.

Clearly, at the extremes of immaturity the worker is passive, dependent on instructions and works erratically and without self-motivation. This may be perceived as the way the nursing care assistants are behaving at the moment with regard to the morning's work; however the problems may be more with their lack of leadership than with their lack of self-motivation.

Giving consideration to Argyris' continuum in the scenario, the nursing assistants may state the following problems in regard to the morning's workload:

- work attitude – they will do whatever is requested of them;
- dependence – they want to be told the priorities;
- behaviour – they don't recognise the importance of client dignity;
- interests – they lack professionalism;
- concern – they aren't concerned where clients eat their meals;
- position – they are too junior to influence practice;
- self-awareness – they don't feel able to voice their opinions.

Clearly, with this set of values, the nursing assistants are not going to work in a structured and priority-led fashion, but instead respond to 'whoever shouts loudest' and this might not be a client.

One of the last writers on leadership, who only considered the individual rather than the situation, was Herzberg (1966, cited by La Monica, 1994), whose work reflects Maslow's hierarchy of needs. He felt that *hygiene factors* such as pay, working conditions and poor job security demotivated staff, as found in Maslow's lower-level needs. In the scenario, the nursing care assistants may feel that the change of home ownership and designation from residential to nursing status has been detrimental to them. They may well feel that bringing in more registered nurses will lead to job losses or pay cuts.

Herzberg points out, however, that it is not simply the reverse situation – high pay, good working conditions and job security – that motivate staff. Instead the *motivators* reflect the higher levels of Maslow's hierarchy, where achievement, recognition, responsibility, the work itself and personal or professional growth lead to self-actualisation.

Kim as a manger clearly believes that you and Nicky are self-motivated, and you have already demonstrated that you are not McGregor's theory X workers. You perform well because it is not Herzberg hygiene factors that are driving you to change practice, but self-motivation and professional accountability; you demonstrate maturity in Argyris' view. You are aware that even if the positive traits apply to you and Nicky, they may well not apply to other members of the workforce. Patience may well be very concerned about her 'hygiene factors' and so refuses the leadership role.

Activity 4.4   *Reflection*

Reflect on an incident at home or work when you did something well but didn't get the recognition for it that you believed was due. How did you feel? Or perhaps you can remember a time when a task was so boring that even if you were being paid, you couldn't be bothered to do it.

As this is a personal reflection, no outline answer is given.

This activity should make you think about how difficult it can be to remain motivated when the work is boring, or you never receive praise from your colleagues. Overall a little praise goes a long way in maintaining motivation and costs nothing.

Styles of leadership in change

The model of leadership utilised for changing the medicines management aspect is part of the 1960s model of Lewin et al. (Marquis and Huston, 2006). Their research identified three very different leadership styles. The authors were educational psychologists who considered how children interacted when asked to perform a task. If the children were given instruction in what to do by the *authoritarian* leader, they accomplished the task successfully as they followed the leader's directions. In future situations the children needed either more direction or developed their own forceful leader who imposed his or her will and direction.

In the *laissez-faire* led group, leadership was missing; the group did what it wanted; the children were not shown how best to achieve a task. There was no direction from the leader, no discussion or guidance and ultimately the children neither learnt how to work together nor achieved the task.

In the *democratic* group, the leader encouraged discussion, the sharing of ideas, an emphasis on we, not I, and decision-making that is effective. The children learnt to share ideas and target problems as a team, working together with a supportive helpful leader. In future tasks this group of children demonstrated how they had learnt to work together with appropriate and agreed leadership, to achieve tasks; hence many view the democratic leadership style as best.

All three styles do have a place in healthcare settings today, although generally the leader who has a democratic style may well be preferred routinely. In an emergency situation the authoritarian and directive approach can ensure efficient activities with an established clear goal. The laissez-faire approach is a particularly useful leadership style when creativity is needed; it works best when equals from different backgrounds come together on a project.

A number of other writers during the latter part of the twentieth century have considered the way staff and management interact to get tasks achieved. Overall there has been recognition that the interplay between staff and leader (or manager) is key to effective outcomes in the workplace, but that the task and situation may affect this. Schein (1970, cited by Marquis and Huston, 2006, p53) described *how the relationship between the leader's personality and the specific situation* affected the outcome. This interactional or systems theory led to the development of more theories and proposals on how staff and leaders should interact for maximum effectiveness. Burns (1978, cited by Marquis and Huston, 2006) first proposed the *transactional* leader, the manager concerned with day-to-day tasks and outcomes, and the *transformational* leader, empowering and visionary.

Scenario

In the nursing home the new medicines administration system is rapidly implemented and, when challenged about the new procedures, all of you say that this change is vital to comply with legislation and prevent accidents, hence you act as transactional leaders. In due course the changes are accepted and become standard practice.

The way that the morning's workload is completed is a less tangible problem with a range of possible solutions, so an autocratic leader would not be effective. It is also clear that the laissez-faire approach, of letting the staff do as they want every morning, has not achieved appropriate outcomes. So Nicky suggests a democratic approach, getting the staff involved with what they need to do; you argue that the staff don't seem to have the same vision as yourselves. Nicky's exasperation with the current situation shows, when at the staff meeting she asks why the nursing care assistants aren't committed to getting everyone appropriately ready for lunch. You think that they need to commit to an 'ideal of care'. You want to give them a vision of exemplary care, to transform the way they think about the clients and you are thus a transformational leader.

You and Nicky decide that one lunch time next week, as you need some time to get organised, you will 'play a trick' in the staff room where everyone is eating. You will act out some of the 'problems' that you perceive are happening and see what results. Patience and Kim are again left 'holding the fort' and now Patience is as passionate as you and Nicky are about getting the changes in place: she is no longer concerned about losing her job (Herzberg's hygiene factors have been resolved).

So on cue you are pushed into the staff room in your night clothes on a commode. Everyone looks up and stares at you both. Someone asks if it is charity fund-raising fancy dress, to which of course you just say no. Nicky passes you your lunch tray and tells everyone else to carry on eating. She also puts a urinal on the table, albeit full of plain water, and starts to leave the staff room.

continued . . .

Some of the staff laugh nervously; others get up to leave but Nicky stops them. The atmosphere has changed and you know the shock tactics have disturbed the status quo. (This is the *unfreeze* first step in Lewin's change theory.)

Nicky returns and asks everyone why they are so shocked by your behaviour: after all, this happens all the time in the client areas, and the staff reluctantly agree that it does. You ask what everyone felt about seeing this behaviour in their dining room and why they were disturbed by it. Then you ask them to write down their concerns on sticky notes before they go back to work. Once you have the ideas on paper you prepare to leave the room, but reiterate to everyone to think on what they have just seen.

Activity 4.5   *Evidence-based practice and research*

Have you ever witnessed an aspect of care that conflicts with practice that you believed to be correct? What should you do?

An outline answer is provided at the end of the chapter.

The leaders in the scenario are behaving in different ways depending on the changes that they want to implement. In the medicines management part, a transactional or autocratic leadership style is needed to ensure that necessary changes are implemented without delay. In this part there are no decisions to be made, no alternatives to the proposed safe practice and the leadership is situational.

However, in planning a better way of managing the workload in the morning, it is vital that everyone accepts and works towards a similar goal. The shock tactics were designed to provide a visual stimulus to change and to inspire a new vision of good care. This is transformational leadership and requires a democratic style which engages and listens to all the team members.

Contingency theories of leadership, such as those of Fiedler (1974, cited by Girvin, 1998), propose that the leader's influence depends on three variables: the leader's relationship with subordinates, the leader's formal power and the task to be achieved. In this leadership model Fiedler suggests that some leaders are task-oriented and some are relationship-oriented and that in difficult situations the second style may be more successful. Overall, the leader needs to be flexible and responsive to the task to be achieved and the needs of the workforce. Victor Vroom's (1964, cited by Girvin, 1998) work might be seen to identify the foundation of both transactional and transformational leadership (Table 4.2). He recognised the need for the task to be understood by the workers, as well as the workers' own goals to be met.

Transactional leader	Transformational leader
Focuses on management tasks	Identifies common values
Is a caretaker, temporary	Is committed, for the long haul
Uses trade-offs to meet goals	Inspires others with vision
Does not identify shared values	Has long-term vision
Examines causes	Looks at effects
Uses contingency reward	Empowers others

Table 4.2. Transactional and transformational leadership
Source: Marquis and Huston (2006), p56.

Scenario

As the changes to the medicines management are settling down, you and Nicky start to tackle the morning workload chaos by first looking at the comments on the sticky notes. It is clear that many of the staff also perceive the morning to be chaotic and would like direction in better ways of working. Some of them also comment on your role play: *made me think about what I do every day*! and *where has dignity gone*? You are both pleased about this type of comment as it is the first step to getting things changed; however comments such as *the patients don't know what's going on around here anyway* are of much more concern. So you meet again with Kim, the home manager, to discuss your plans.

It seems that fundamentally no client is cared for by the same person in any one week; this was a fall-back from the residential home days when some clients clearly needed nursing care and were much more demanding on staff time. This has changed: there are more nursing needs, but also there are more staff and, with more having permanent contracts, there is less reliance on agency carers. So, using a transformational leadership style, you all agree on a variety of ways forward, firstly identifying a common set of values agreed by all the staff: anyone who can't agree to this will be asked to leave the home. You want all the staff to acknowledge that the care they provide would meet their own standards if they were to become a client at the home.

The philosophy of care is that the residents will have dignity, privacy and safety in a homely environment.

Second, you divide the clients into two teams, each led by a staff nurse. Any other trained nurses on at the same time as the team lead will act as support as and where required that day. The workload of the clients is assessed and each assigned to one of the teams. You all recognise that this will mean that at first the teams are working in an apparently ad hoc way throughout the home, as each team will have clients in each wing. It is agreed that as any client leaves the home and a bed becomes available, there will be an attempt to move the existing or new clients into the appropriate team wing, if they are willing to move 'home'.

continued . . .

This is part of the long-term strategy to facilitate easier ways of working, as the staff will start to understand each client's needs and meet those needs more quickly and effectively.

Third, the mid-morning coffee break will be staggered and be taken by everyone, at appropriate times, so that no one is left alone without support.

Finally, Kim has agreed to hold monthly staff meetings during working hours (staff will be paid if off duty) to discuss all issues and concerns. These meetings will be an hour long, with an agenda, and subsequent minutes and action plans.

This transformational leadership style will improve care as well as job satisfaction.

By improving the way the staff work in the home and their job satisfaction, the overall quality of nursing care will improve and, coupled with the changes to medicines management, there should be less risk of harm to clients. If transformational leadership empowers the staff towards the organisational goals of choice then it is also important that on a day-to-day basis problems are dealt with speedily and efficiently by a transactional manager. Kim recognises that both Nicky and you will make rational nursing decisions, which she will support, but that you will rapidly refer organisational problems to her for action.

Emotional intelligence in leadership

Most recently writers have recognised that a key requirement of effective leaders is *emotional intelligence,* the ability to understand the emotions in themselves and their staff and to manage it towards the organisational goal. Vitello-Cicciu (2007) writes further about this concept and how this translates into nursing care situations as well as organisational ones. The nurse needs to consider the patient's perception of the situation when managing complex situations. Leaders should be alert to the development of misunderstandings and poor communication between different 'cultures' of the organisation, to be a *cultural bridge* and to step in to manage this effectively (de Ruiter and Saphiere, 2001, cited by Marquis and Huston, 2006) . Finally, Porter-O'Grady (2003) wrote about how in times of change it can be very difficult to ensure that leadership, accountability, vision and empowerment are developing as fast. The terms 'leadership' and 'management' have many similarities and differences but both must work to achieve the organisation's goals.

Activities: brief outline answers

Activity 4.2

You must bring any concerns you have about care to your employer in the first instance and then to the regulatory bodies, such as the NMC, the CQC or the police depending on the seriousness of the problem. You always remain accountable for your actions to your clients.

Activity 4.3

It is likely that you will have seen the ward drug trolley, a shared locked cupboard in places like accident and emergency or the intensive treatment unit and possibly patients with their own locked cupboards. What is important is the security of the medication in a public place and safe administration to the correct client. Identification of clients in their own 'home' such as a nursing home can be difficult when they quite reasonably don't wear name bands. However you should always feel confident that you can identify patients through their photograph or other means rather than relying on junior colleagues.

Activity 4.5

This activity may have made you think about a different way of providing wound care, such as the clean technique for managing a chronic venous leg ulcer or non-sterile intermittent self-catheterisation. As a student in a hospital setting you will have been taught that wound care and catheterisations are both aseptic procedures, yet you will have seen something very different in these situations.

There are various ways to tackle differences in practice. The first and simplest is to ask directly why a certain activity is being performed in a particular way. If this answer is not helpful or your query is dismissed as irrelevant, then do a little investigative work yourself in books or online, as there may be some useful explanations. If your queries still can't be addressed then go to a senior colleague or line manager to see if he or she can provide information or rationale. If you feel that the practice is clearly unsafe or puts patients or staff at risk, you should write an incident report form so that it can be actioned further.

Further reading and useful websites

ebooks.adelaide.edu.au/m/machiavelli/niccolo/m149p/

Try reading the original text of **Machiavelli's** *The Prince*, translated into English by WK Marriott.

www.mindtools.com/pages/article/newLDR_84.htm

This is a good source on leadership and other managerial skills.

Chapter 5
Taking on a mentorship role

NMC Standards for Pre-registration Nursing Education

This chapter will address the following competencies:

Domain 1: Professional values

1. All nurses must practise with confidence according to *The code: Standards of conduct, performance and ethics for nurses and midwives* (NMC 2008), and within other recognised ethical and legal frameworks. They must be able to recognise and address ethical challenges relating to people's choices and decision-making about their care, and act within the law to help them and their families and carers find acceptable solutions.

Domain 4: Leadership, management and team working

5. All nurses must facilitate nursing students and others to develop their competence, using a range of professional and personal development skills.

NMC Essential Skills Clusters

This chapter will address the following ESCs:

Cluster: Care, compassion and communication

5. People can trust the newly registered graduate nurse to engage with them in a warm, sensitive and compassionate way.

By entry to register

13. Through reflection and evaluation demonstrates commitment to personal and professional development and life-long learning.

Cluster: Organisational aspects of care

12. People can trust the newly registered graduate nurse to respond to their feedback and a wide range of other sources to learn, develop and improve services.

By entry to register

8. As an individual team member and team leader, actively seeks and learns from feedback to enhance care and own and others' professional development.

Introduction

This chapter is about supporting students in a learning environment. It will discuss the shift from being a trainee to being trainer, in light of the NMC Standards for Pre-registration Nursing Education (NMC, 2010). The scenarios are based on experience in an outpatient department (OPD) setting, where the nurse is also learning her own specialist skills.

Scenario

Since you started working in the OPD, you have noticed how many learning opportunities exist; however you are aware that, as a student, you always thought this would be a boring place to work. It was not your first choice of job on qualifying six months ago, but it was the only post available and the benefits of working close to home and Monday to Friday have also helped you settle in. Recently the departmental manager (Clive) has suggested that, rather than having students on 'day trips' from other areas, they should have a student placed in the OPD full time. Some of your colleagues don't think this placement would be suitable and others state they haven't the time to manage a student, but you think they are missing a golden opportunity. The OPD has clinics of every conceivable medical speciality, as well as many that are run solely by nurses, and you know that many of the staff, both medical and nursing, enjoy explaining their work. As new member of staff you have found yourself back in student mode as you learnt both your job and about the specialities having clinics here. The departmental manager and the senior sister (Annie) in the clinics have approached you, because you are only recently qualified, to set up a working party to look at the issues involved.

Subsequently a meeting is set up with you, the senior sister, one other staff nurse (Irene) and a member of the local university academic staff (Jacky) to look at the issues involved in more detail. The sister introduces everyone and sets a timescale for what she describes as a task and finish group. Task and finish groups typically come together to manage a particular task in a set timeframe and then disband, and each participant has an equal voice in the group's objectives. In this case the university academic explains what will be needed in order to prepare the area as a student placement and the objective of receiving a first-year student in six months' time.

Jacky explains what is required from a practice placement and this includes preparation of the mentor and buddy mentors, the educational audit, but because the OPD is part of the

continued . . .

trust a workplace agreement will already exist. (This is the legal agreement between the higher-education institution and any placement provider.) Irene asks what is meant by an educational audit, as she has never heard of it, and Jacky explains that it is part of the quality framework. She also states that the team will need to consider what educational opportunities exist in OPD and perhaps work out a learning plan for the proposed eight-week placement.

When you were a student you may have had little idea of how carefully areas are prepared in order for them to have students and may even have felt that no one really cared what happened. First, areas that are going to have students require an educational audit for their suitability (NMC, 2004); this is a process where the area's learning opportunities and student support mechanisms are identified. The trust or the organisation's senior managers will also have to sign a legal contract with the university to identify the requirements of both parties and this fits within a nationally agreed framework (Department of Health, 2006).

The university will want to know who will directly support the student on placement and complete the necessary practice assessment documents.

Activity 5.1   *Reflection*

Think back to your practice placements during your training. Was there an area in which you learnt more or less than you expected before you started? Was there one which was more enjoyable than expected? Why do you think this happened?

As this is a personal reflection, no outline answer is given.

In the activity you may have recalled how you did have preconceived ideas about a placement after hearing gossip. You may have worked on some very busy and demanding areas, yet your mentor made all possible learning opportunities open to you.

Lifelong learning

Scenario

The discussion in the meeting moves along to the issue of student support and the role of the mentor and/or assessor (NMC, 2008a). You anticipated that it would automatically be the sister and are surprised to hear your name mentioned. However Sister Annie explains that, although she would really like to work directly with a student, this is not really feasible, particularly as the student is a first-year. The academic, Jacky, who will be the unit's link with the university to support learners, discusses why the Sister would not be best suited

continued . . .

and also explains the need for you to undergo formal mentorship training to be fully prepared to support a learner. She also explains that a space on such a module (course) is currently available, starting in a fortnight's time. You ask why Irene, the other staff nurse, who has been qualified longer than you, isn't the first choice for the course. It seems she was, but unfortunately she has annual leave booked over the first three days of the course and as such could not complete the work. She comments that it has been agreed that she will attend the next available course and that she will work as your buddy mentor with the first student. Sister Annie asks if you would be happy to undertake the course and the associated assignment; much to your own surprise, you say yes. On reflection you know that after a nine-month gap from your last pre-registration assignment you actually miss studying, something you'd never believed possible as you battled the third-year assignments!

The NMC (2008a) expects nurses to have been qualified for at least a year before acting as mentors, and so by the time the student arrives, this criterion will have been met. Annie explains that, as she already holds a teaching qualification, she will support and assess you with your mentorship training and be a resource when the student arrives. Jacky is able to present you with a course handbook before she leaves the meeting and Sister Annie suggests that you might look at the practical learning and teaching tasks required in advance of the programme. You leave the meeting excited and optimistic about making the OPD a great learning environment.

Lifelong learning is one of the government and healthcare employers' objectives, to try to ensure that employees and staff keep up to date with current working practices. In *Liberating the NHS: Developing the healthcare workforce* (Department of Health, 2010a), the government recognised that *60% of the staff currently working in the NHS will probably still be delivering healthcare in ten years' time* (p23), referring to the need to update staff already employed rather than just focusing on the education of those entering the health service. Lifelong learning isn't just about formal taught courses – it is a philosophy that engages staff throughout their careers. The EU Commission in 2000 defined lifelong learning as *all learning activity undertaken throughout life, with the aim of improving knowledge, skills and competence within a civic, social and/or employment related perspective.*

It is frequently a surprise to ex-students that in a relatively short timeframe they start to miss studying and having academic goals. Staff may find themselves looking for further studies in a particular clinical field or in more general education or management. It is really important that these aspirations are met, even though financial constraints appear to act against any formal education. There has thus been a move away from face-to-face teaching on day-release post-registration to e-learning or distance-learning formats, which staff can undertake in their leisure time at home. Whatever method is used, nurses are obliged under post-registration education and practice guidelines (NMC, 2011) to ensure that they attend a minimum of 35 hours' study over three years. (They must also work for at least 450 hours over three years, in a capacity reliant on NMC registration.) This would be expected to be above and beyond any mandatory updates set up by the employer.

Mentorship training and preparation are clearly defined by the NMC (2008a), which sets standards for the education of staff in practice working with learners. The university and its practice placement providers have to reassure the NMC that when they provide under graduate pre-registration training, sufficient effort has been made to support learners while on placement. The Health Professions Council (2009) also recognises the importance of having suitably prepared clinical educators, although they may not use the term 'mentor'.

Mentorship in action

Scenario

As the meeting progresses you start to realise the level of your responsibilities towards any student placed with you, but are reassured by the others that you are up to the challenge and that they will support you. Sister Annie has said that undertaking your mentorship training will actually put you back into the learner mode and that she will be assessing you during the course. Annie is an experienced member of staff, who undertook learning about educational theory when she was working in community as a district nurse and has a wide experience of supporting learners in various contexts. Although happy about undertaking the theory component of the mentorship education you wonder out loud who will be your learner prior to the student coming on placement? Jacky, the academic link tutor, says that any learner will be appropriate and that it doesn't have to be a pre-registration student, and Clive, the departmental manager, comments that a new healthcare assistant (HCA), Marie, will be joining the ward next week and that she will provide an ideal learner. With both the availability of a 'captive' learner and a place on the mentorship module, you start to look forward to academic studies again.

The manager then mentions that before the educational audit occurs there must be a review of the learning opportunities within the department. Irene explains that she has been thinking about what learning opportunities existed, because she misses working with learners, and was aware of the need to oriente the new HCA and her ideas are committed to paper. Both Sister Annie and Jacky are impressed with the work Irene has undertaken and so you volunteer to help her develop the ideas and commit the material to an electronic orientation package. Jacky asks that any orientation material developed contain not only the clinical resources, but also details about the expertise and additional training of the staff employed within the department. This is so that she can develop the live register of mentors (NMC, 2008a).

Facilitating learning

The mentorship module or course will help prepare you for the role of mentor/assessor and identify tools that will assist with learning and attitudes and behaviours that block learning. The NMC (2008a) *Standards to Support Learning and Assessment in Practice* identify a number of key areas that can either facilitate or detract from learning. The Health Professions Council (2009) has also set standards and these cover similar areas, although they are more generic.

The scenario shows an instant opportunity to undertake mentorship training, but the situation in the real world is likely to be different. You may need to consider face-to-face delivery, which is time-consuming and costly to your employer, compared with delivery through distance or e-learning, at lower cost in your own time. Find out details of the mentorship training on offer with your local higher education institute provider.

No outline answer is provided for this individual activity.

The NMC specifies that students must be in direct or indirect supervision from their mentor for at least 40% of the time, but most educational situations would want this to be higher. For this reason the working environment must be such as to allow student and mentor to work together and not be so busy as to prevent adequate supervision: working with the mentor will be the most productive way to facilitate learning. Having a student working alongside a trained nurse at all times is ideal, but this needs to be managed carefully. It may take longer for any activity to be completed when it is being demonstrated to a learner by the mentor and in some situations this may have a detrimental effect on patient care. If this is the case, then the mentor should explain that she will carry out the nursing intervention by herself and then discuss it with the learner.

Balancing different needs

It is also important that the clinical area recognises how many students, of any kind, that it can reasonably support, to ensure good working relationships. Students must not simply be pairs of hands to help with the work, but despite being supernumerary, students need to and must get involved in day-to-day nursing care. For instance, a student nurse may want to be involved with oral drug administration, but her mentor in the OPD knows that she has a limited knowledge of drug usage or interaction and a ward-based drug round will not occur. So the mentor has to explain that the student must first demonstrate safe understanding and administration of medicines with only one patient rather than the whole unit. The mentor also asks the student to start learning the common usages and complications of the drugs used in a particular OPD eye clinic (in this case, eye drops) and then call on the student to demonstrate her knowledge and understanding by administering that drug, under supervision, to a patient. By learning about one patient's medication the student will be able to relate the use of the drug to the patient's condition and potential side effects. In this way the mentor has both facilitated the student's learning and considered the working environment.

Consider how you could use one medication, frequently used in your working environment, to make a learning experience for a student.

An outline answer is provided at the end of the chapter.

Another way of facilitating learning is for the mentor to discuss with the student her learning needs, and to discuss her existing knowledge and skills. The mentor then helps the student to make use of the opportunities from the clinical area to meet the learner's set objectives or practice assessments. Junior learners often don't know where to focus their learning and the use of a student's assessment material or the unit's orientation pack may help with this. In the OPD there will be a number of clinics which have different patient situations and many different professionals will work there. Understanding the roles and functions of other professionals will help student nurses to understand their involvement in the patient journey. This has been recognised by the government and thus the NMC (2008a) and education providers to improve interprofessional learning and working.

From mentor to assessor

It is frequently the situation in clinical areas that the mentor who has supported, guided and empowered the student with learning has also, towards the end of the placement, become the student's assessor. It can be a difficult situation because as the student works alongside the mentor a degree of friendship may develop, which can make judging the student's performance difficult. In order to reduce the difficulties that a friendship might bring, the mentor should ensure that a professional attitude is maintained at all times. Warmth, empathy and understanding are vital skills for a mentor, as these promote learning, but the mentor also needs to set learning objectives and measure performance against these objectives. All workers need feedback on their performance and students, in particular, should have feedback on their performance frequently. Usually feedback occurs in an informal way as care is delivered when the mentor asks the student about knowledge or judges the student's skills. It is thus good practice to review students formatively at a midpoint in a placement, so that if necessary practice can improve, and then summatively at the end (NMC, 2008a). (The higher-education academy defines 'formative' as assessment for learning and 'summative' as assessment of learning: **www.heacademy.ac.uk/ assets/cebe/Documents/projects/innovativeprojects/Effective_and_Efficient_ Methods_of_Formative_Assessment.pdf**.) As the mentor/assessor you are in an ideal position to develop good practice and challenge poor practice; however, many mentors do find being constructively critical difficult and they find failing a student even harder. Experienced staff both in the clinical area and from the university will always support a mentor in a difficult situation, to ensure that you are following due process. 'Failing to fail' is a concept explored by Duffy (2003) in her seminal work for the NMC, when she considered why mentors/assessors allowed incompetent students to complete their practice placements successfully; this work has subsequently been influential in guiding mentor preparation.

Activity 5.4   *Communication*

Access a copy of Duffy's work (see references and Further study, at the end of this chapter). You could also read articles on the same topic. Consider whether you would have difficulty failing an incompetent student.

As this is a personal reflection, no outline answer is supplied.

Learning styles

As a mentor you need to try to understand how another individual learns, as it may be different from how you learn. Honey and Mumford (1982) considered that there were four ways that individuals learn best and that teaching strategies should consider this (Learning Styles Questionnaire, 2012).

Theory summary: Honey and Mumford learning styles

Activists are 'hands-on' learners and prefer to have a go and learn through trial and error.
Reflectors are 'tell me' learners and prefer to be thoroughly briefed before proceeding.
Theorists are 'convince me' learners and want reassurance that a project makes sense.
Pragmatists are 'show me' learners and want a demonstration from an acknowledged expert.

Activity 5.5   *Evidence-based practice and research*

Research more into Honey and Mumford's work. Now undertake a personal learning-style assessment so that you can consider how to work with learners. Honey and Mumford's work is available online and is copyright-protected.

An outline answer is provided at the end of the chapter.

You may recognise, when looking at learning styles, the way mentors have treated you or others in some of the comments Duffy makes. Reflection on these styles will help you plan learning opportunities. For instance, your learner may like to get involved as an activist and learn in a hands-on way, but you prefer a more cautious approach, being a reflector. Clearly it may not be possible to choose a student who has the same kind of learning style as yourself, but an understanding of the different learning styles should help you as a mentor to consider how best to develop knowledge and skills and accommodate different learning styles.

You cannot work with your learner all the time. A mentor should also consider how to make the best use of any leaning opportunities, and how to support the student, in their absence. The use of a mentor and buddy or co-mentor may well facilitate this. Typically the mentor and buddy discuss with the student what experiences and learning can take place in the mentor's absence. The NMC (2008a) emphasises the importance of both leadership and good working relationships in the mentoring process.

It is also vitally important that students should be exposed to care which is delivered using an evidence-based approach and which follows due policy and procedure. The educational audit (NMC, 2004) is a way of capturing the interests and additional qualifications of all the staff on a unit. The knowledge and skills of all the staff in any area should be available to the student as a learning resource, although the timing may need careful consideration.

From specific skills to general knowledge

Scenario

A few days later you and the new HCA, Marie, are rostered to work together and as it is her first day you introduce yourself and start showing her the layout of the OPD. Unfortunately there isn't a map and no easy way to find your way around the whole building. (Patients and clients have less trouble, as they are told to follow certain coloured routes taped to the floor, guiding them from one area to another as care dictates.) So you decide to obtain a floor plan from the building department and identify the functional areas; this will make sense as part of the orientation package for all new staff. You realise how much you have learnt in six months and how an area like the OPD could be very challenging to a shy new staff member. Marie is such a person; she has not worked as an HCA before and has spent the last few weeks on an induction programme to the trust, which has provided her with some baseline skills. Marie is keen to learn but is clearly intimidated by any medical staff, even when they mean well. You reassure her that in the OPD everyone's role is vital and the patient is the most important. It is clear that mentoring Marie will provide you with a useful experience and help with your formal mentoring course, although you are aware of the different roles and responsibilities of the HCA and the student.

One area that Marie has to undertake is urine testing for patients attending any OPD appointment. You have decided that this is one of the activities that you could help her with and which might tick some of the mentorship course requirements. Marie states that she's seen urine testing done and it looks easy, so you suggest that it actually requires more knowledge and skills than she thinks, particularly to ensure that she follows safe practice. As such, you introduce her to both the *Marsden Manual* (Dougherty and Lister, 2011) and the trust's own intranet, which can provide her with the practical details of all the tasks needed in clinical practice. As a member of staff Marie can get access to the trust intranet and library, but you wonder what students have to do and decide to find out. Several patients later you are happy that Marie can test urine on her own in a safe and professional manner; and on reflection it surprises you how much information you have covered for such an apparently simple task. You have treated Marie as a learner regardless of her status; you have asked about her existing experiences with urine testing, and then considered what knowledge, skills and attitudes are required for this routine task. Most importantly, you believe that you have convinced Marie that it is good to ask questions and that if she needs help and reassurance in any activity she only has to ask.

Testing urine seems a simple task which is frequently carried out but it can be used by the clever mentor to introduce a range of topics to the learner, covering all aspects of knowledge, skills and attitudes and specific parts of the Essential Skills Cluster (NMC, 2011):

- privacy and dignity when asking a patient to produce a urine sample (attitude) (ESC 2);
- the appropriate use of personal protective equipment when dealing with body fluids (knowledge) (ESC 22);
- the correct use of the testing equipment (skills) (ESC 20);
- the rationale for testing urine and the significance of the findings (knowledge) (ESC 6);
- documenting appropriately and informing others (skills and attitude) (ESC 10).

Activity 5.6   *Team working*

Next time you have a new or relatively inexperienced learner, try to teach all aspects of urine testing. If you really attempt to cover all the opportunities to learn through routine urine testing you will be surprised at how many areas of safe practice can be explored.

An outline answer is provided at the end of the chapter.

Scenario

Not all the staff seem to like working with learners and yet you know that the *Code of Conduct* (NMC, 2008b) identifies the responsibilities of all registered nurses to assist in the learning process. It doesn't offer an opt-out clause, and you are also aware that the trust's staff grading structure puts an emphasis on peer support and continuing education for all. You notice that some staff behave differently towards you when you are working with Marie, in her learning capacity. You realise that they feel that you will not be able to carry your workload if you help with Marie's learning. You can't understand this view: it seems very short-sighted of them, as Marie will be a useful asset to the team, providing she is offered some teaching and leadership in the first instance, after which she will grow in independence and competence.

You have now given more thought to supporting Marie in a constructive fashion and how this might be similar to a first-year student. As you attend the mentorship training you are asked to look at the local university's student assessment document as well as the NMC requirements. The new curriculum will be slightly different to that on which you studied, but there are lots of similarities as well as differences. You are pleased to see the emphasis on numeracy and wonder how you can develop Marie's skills in this area, as she won't be undertaking medicines management (ESC 36; NMC, 2010). In the OPD one important task for HCAs is the accurate recording and documentation of height and weight measurement as well as pulse, temperature and blood pressure. The department has returned to the use of manual equipment for monitoring vital signs and so this is to be the focus of much of your mentoring. These skills will also apply to first-year students, although they may be involved with some of the prescribed dressing treatments or medications administered as well.

continued . . .

As time progresses, Marie develops in her HCA role and becomes an asset to the OPD team. Your manager congratulates you on her development and on the teaching session, which you undertook as part of the mentorship module. You are really looking forward to the placement of the first-year student with you and welcome the opportunity to help the student learn.

Delegation

As a mentor it is important that you support your learner constructively and also recognise that some practices can actually damage learning. As a busy member of staff it may seem appropriate to delegate tasks to colleagues, but an effective mentor delegates carefully and gets feedback on process and outcome, not just dumping work on junior colleagues. Morton-Cooper and Palmer (cited by Downie and Basford, 2003) consider the term 'toxic mentor': Such a person hampers learning, and the first type is the 'dumper' who is either not accessible to the learner or doesn't support the learner in new tasks. The 'blocker' refuses requests from the learner which would enhance learning and the 'destroyer/criticiser' undermines the confidence of the learner directly or indirectly.

With Marie you have worked together to use urine testing as a platform for many aspects of nursing; even confidentiality and dignity were discussed in the context of taking the specimen. The correct use of protective equipment and infection control were considered in handling the specimen as well as literacy and professionalism in terms of testing, labelling and recording the specimen.

A very similar process could be used with the student nurse as it is important that activities are broken down into component parts, each of which can be used as a learning activity. If a toxic mentor was working with a learner on urinalysis, such a person would typically demonstrate the procedure once and fail to explain the totality of the activity; or might refuse to let the learner practice for fear of an error; or perhaps would fail to acknowledge that the learner has carried out the procedure correctly. Any of these responses is likely to leave a learner frustrated and the mentor–mentee relationship may break down; however, a good mentor who shows competence and commitment to the role is likely to be rewarded by the development of the learner into a competent practitioner.

All staff need to engage in learning and teaching throughout their careers, and we should always want to participate in these activities.

Activities: brief outline answers

Activity 5.3

As your experience develops so does your knowledge base and you may not even be aware how much you have learnt. So this activity is getting you to think about what you would say to a patient/client or learner if that person asked about a medication.

For instance, take the drug paracetamol:

Knowledge: used as analgesic or antipyretic: used in combination with other analgesics to potentiate effect; complications and overdose risks.

Skills: drug dispensing to avoid contamination of stock; drug calculations to ensure correct dose; careful reading of prescription chart; food hygiene issues.

Attitudes: ascertaining pain level of patient; reviewing effectiveness of analgesia; ensuring that the right patient receives the right dose at the right time; advising patients on self-administration.

Activity 5.5

If you have completed the work suggested by Honey and Mumford on yourself, you should be able to recognise how your own learning style may be different from a learner placed with you. As a mentor you need to consider your learner's needs rather than your own.

Activity 5.6

Urine testing might seem like a simple and repetitive task but break it down using Bloom's taxonomy (see Further study, below):

Knowledge: why urine is tested; different types of urine test; what can be identified from the results.

Skills: taking the right sample at the right time of day; putting the sample in the correct receptacle/specimen bottle; safe labelling; infection control issues and personal protective clothing.

Attitudes: approaching the client; maintain confidentiality; dealing with the findings professionally; reporting findings and documentation.

Further reading and useful websites

This will increase your knowledge on mentoring:

Aston, L and Hallam, P (2011) *Successful Mentoring in Nursing*. Exeter: Learning Matters.

www.nwlink.com/~donclark/hrd/bloom.html

Bloom's taxonomy of learning domains.

www.dh.gov.uk/en/Publicationsandstatistics/Publications/PublicationsPolicyAndGuidance/DH_4133085

Here the Department of Health website explains the agreements between placement organisations and higher-education institutes. It sets out the whole contract and the requirements to support learners.

Dougherty, L and Lister, S (eds) (2011) *The Royal Marsden Hospital Manual of Clinical Nursing Procedures*, 8th edition. **www.royalmarsdenmanual.com/view/online.html**

Downie, C and Basford, P (2003) *Mentoring in Practice: A reader*. London: University of Greenwich.

Duffy, K (2004) Mentors need more support to fail incompetent students *British Journal of Nursing*, 113(10):582. Commentary (with reference) on her research at: **shsmentor.swan.ac.uk/Documents/6%20Failing%20to%20Fail%2024%2009%2008/entries%20in%20text/NMC.pdf**

Duffy, K (2004) *Failing Students*. London: Nursing and Midwifery Council.

Chapter 6
Risks and decisions

NMC Standards for Pre-registration Nursing Education

This chapter will address the following competencies:

Domain 1: Professional values

4. All nurses must work in partnership with service users, carers, families, groups, communities and organisations. They must manage risk, and promote health and wellbeing while aiming to empower choices that promote self-care and safety.

Domain 3: Nursing practice and decision-making

7. All nurses must be able to recognise and interpret signs of normal and deteriorating mental and physical health and respond promptly to maintain or improve the health and comfort of the service user, acting to keep them and others safe.

NMC Essential Skills Clusters

This chapter will address the following ESCs:

Cluster: Infection prevention and control

21. People can trust the newly registered graduate nurse to identify and take effective measures to prevent and control infection in accordance with local and national policies.

By entry to register

11. Recognises infection risk and reports and acts in situations where there is need for health promotion and protection and public health strategies.

Chapter aims

After reading this chapter, you will be able to:

*   describe a risk assessment;
*   manage risks to people through reduction and containment;
*   practise decision-making and delegation in areas of risk;
*   manage risks to the clinical environment.

Introduction

This chapter will have a focus on untoward incidents such as a potential methicillin-resistant *Staphylococcus aureus* (MRSA) infection or drug error and sets the scenario in an elder-care ward. The importance of risk assessment, reduction and containment will be covered, as well as decision-making and delegation. The links to quality assurance will be discussed in relationship to standards and policies.

Being a leader in some situations may seem to be quite easy, particularly if the workforce or your colleagues are happy to implement or adapt to the rapid changes found in the workplace. However, in other situations you may well wish that you had no decision-making responsibilities and that it was always easy to 'switch off' when you leave work. For many managers, leading the team may not be as difficult as getting the task done alone, when the staff situation seems stacked against you. The scenario in this chapter will consider how you manage a junior member of the nursing team, who doesn't want to comply with the rules of infection control.

Managing risks to people

Scenario

You have been in post as a staff nurse on the elder-care unit for ten months; you have finished your six-month preceptorship period and have now become team leader for one group, the red team (to identify the different teams, your team is known by a colour, but other forms of identification might be by a letter or team leader's name). You hadn't expected this to happen so quickly as many of your friends, who were also on the trust-wide preceptorship programme, are acting as second in command in a team rather than as leader. Your ward manager has apologised for this rapid rise in seniority, but as you are aware the whole elder-care directorate has been in upheaval as a new ward was opened. St Alfred's Hospital is part of a geographically widespread community trust which made the decision to centralise some elder-care services on the site. With funds raised by the League of Friends, one new ward has recently been refurnished and reopened as an elderly mentally infirm unit. Although the trust was able to appoint some new staff, many of those employed on the other wards at St Alfred's took the opportunity to apply to move areas. In particular those who were mental health-trained have moved across, leaving your ward rather depleted in experience. Your ward manager has tried to reassure you that she and the directorate manager believe you are capable of leading the team, but you have reservations.

The ward manager has recognised that you can't be a mentor for any students on your team, as you have not been qualified for a year (NMC, 2008a), but expects you to act as buddy mentor. This is clearly far from ideal and you can remember how difficult it felt as a student when the designated mentor wasn't around. Still, with that thought in mind, you

continued . . .

hope you will be able to be an effective buddy mentor. It is thus quite a shock to you when you find that all your leadership skills are needed not with the student nurse, but with one of the experienced healthcare assistants (HCAs).

The problem first appears one weekend when you are leading your team. On duty with you are Katy, another staff nurse who qualified last month and has yet to get her PIN (registration with the NMC), two HCAs and a student. The team are responsible for up to 15 patients, who vary in nursing dependency but have mostly been inpatients for some days. Two clients are awaiting discharge to nursing homes once beds become available; six clients are in various stages of stroke rehabilitation; four are recovering from chest or urine infections; one is terminally ill and you have two empty beds. You never like empty beds, particularly at weekends, as the admissions may not be appropriate.

After handover from the night staff, you first ask your team members which patients they would specifically like to care for; this encourages self-motivation and is more satisfying for both patients and staff. (The ward operates team nursing, which provides some continuity of care for the patients and staff; each new admission is assessed for care needs and then allocated to one of the two teams so that the workload is equitable.) The student will come with you, as you are her buddy mentor, on the morning drug round once you have both rapidly greeted all your clients. The rest of the team will get their clients and yours ready for breakfast. It is well established on the ward that meal times are important for client well-being and everyone participates with meals and feeding patients (Department of Health, 2010b). By 11.00 the overall client care seems to be progressing well and all the staff have taken short coffee breaks, so you are relaxing into your managerial role.

Since the scenario raises the issue of drug rounds, now is a good time to look again at the codes of practice which apply to this important aspect of nursing.

Activity 6.1   *Evidence-based practice and research*

What are the local and national issues associated with drug administration?

An outline answer is provided at the end of the chapter.

In the scenario so far, the team has clearly demonstrated that in routine situations they work in a particular way; this is likely to be due to good leadership from the ward manager. As a transformational leader she will have established a vision for the way the unit functions and this will continue even in her absence, as it has become the norm. Some managers are only concerned with the way the staff in their organisation feel, and will do everything to keep them happy. At the other extreme some are only interested in getting the work done, regardless of staff feelings or concerns. This is illustrated diagrammatically as a window with four panes and specifically identified axes, the best managers balancing the needs of the staff with the requirements of the work. In the Ohio State Model of Leadership (Bass and Stogdill, 1990, cited by La Monica Rigolosi, 2005, p87), the axes are labelled 'initiating structures' and 'consideration' and this describes a style of leadership. A leader strong on the 'initiating' axis directs the staff in all aspects of the task and one strong on 'consideration' uses discussion and two-way communication to agree a means of getting the task done. Hersey and Blanchard (1989) modified the grid so that one axis was 'relational behaviour' and one was 'situational behaviour.' Clearly the ideal leader is one who manages to juggle both behavioural and situational considerations to a satisfactory conclusion.

Blake and Mouton (1985), in their leadership grid, took this one stage further when they considered how the leader balanced concern for production over concern for people, with a central point where there is a balance between getting the work done and maintaining the morale of the workforce. In the scenario, as team leader you are showing concern for both the clients' care (the task or production) and concern for people (or relationships) as the work load is progressing at an acceptable pace and staff have had a coffee break. You are thus demonstrating Blake and Mouton's 'organisational man management' performance.

Activity 6.2   *Team working*

Have you ever been in a situation where the task was seen to be so important that individual views or needs were overruled? What did it feel like?

An outline answer is provided at the end of the chapter.

Managing risks to the clinical environment

Scenario

Just after 11.00 the phone rings to tell you that Mr Jones is being admitted to your ward direct from his home, by his GP. This is not uncommon practice, as there is a trust-wide arrangement for GPs and some consultant nurses to have 'admitting rights' to particular wards. For the client this has the definite advantage of bypassing long delays in the Emergency Department; however for the ward team routine preparatory tests will not have occurred. In other words, on the Hersey grid, the trust managers have set up a situation where there is strong high-task orientation (the admitted client) but low relationship orientation (the workforce). Knowing from past experience that patients admitted this way are frequently more ill than you are led to believe on the telephone, you designate the yet-to-register staff nurse (Katy) and one of the HCAs (June) to receive Mr Jones on arrival. You feel that you can trust Katy to do her best in the situation and carry out a holistic assessment of his needs, but this is the first shift you have worked with June, who has just started on the ward.

continued . . .

As you suspected, Mr Jones is very ill on arrival and disoriented. Katy explains to you that it appears he has been cared for at home by his elderly wife and his condition was brought to the attention of the GP when the Jones's niece visited. Mr Jones is dehydrated and has a urine infection, several small pressure sores on his sacrum and a leg ulcer. Mr Jones's wife is with him and she explains that he was in hospital six months ago for treatment of the leg ulcer, but that since the hospital treatment had apparently healed the ulcer, the district nurses no longer visit them. You recall that six months ago the trust had a higher than acceptable level of MRSA in the medical unit and so wonder if Mr Jones might be colonised. Fortunately there is a single side room available, so you instruct Katy and all the team to place him there and that they should be extra vigilant with hand-washing until Mr Jones is pronounced MRSA-free. You ask that Katy, with June's help, undertake a comprehensive assessment of Mr Jones.

Much to your surprise, 15 minutes later you see June coming out of Mr Jones's room and going straight into the main ward, still wearing protective clothing and gloves. So you hurry after her to talk to her about infection control, only to find that she has already gone into the clean utility room, apparently to get a specimen bottle as she is now sorting through the drawers. You call to her and ask her to stop what she is doing and dispose of her contaminated gloves. She turns, says she is in a hurry, and having found what she wants, walks straight past you back to Mr Jones's room.

Activity 6.3   *Evidence-based practice and research*

In the scenario, what issues of poor infection control are in evidence?

An outline answer is provided at the end of the chapter.

As the leader of the team it is necessary to delegate staff to particular tasks and to expect a certain level of responsibility from them. Obviously you don't know much about June's experience, but it is reasonable to assume that as an established employee of the trust she will have had mandatory training on infection control during her employment. Unfortunately attendance at mandatory training doesn't always translate into understanding and compliance with recommended good practice. ('Mandatory' in this setting doesn't mean a legal obligation but rather an obligation between employer and employee.) However, even if June could remember nothing about infection control, she was working with Katy, who should have a good working knowledge of the prevention of cross-contamination and should have been able to remind her.

> ### Scenario
>
> Once June and Katy have completed the assessment of Mr Jones you ask to see them briefly in the ward office, closing the door as they come in. You ask June why she didn't wash her hands or remove the gloves appropriately when leaving the patient. June just shrugs her shoulders and gets her mobile phone out, muttering that she hates working here. Katy remains silent and so as it is midshift you rapidly remind them both about hand-washing and the appropriate use of protective clothing. You state that you'd like to talk to them both again at the end of the shift, once you have all handed over care to other staff.

As a manager, you need to try to tackle problem issues as soon as possible and not allow them to go unchallenged, but you also need to ensure that the workload is completed. This is a classic situation of competing pressures, tackling the poor practice versus the need to care for other patients before lunch time. As you have brought the problem to the attention of the staff immediately, and reminded them of their obligations to prevent cross-infection, you have acted as a transactional leader and been task-focused. At this point it would be easy to believe that your task as a manager has been completed satisfactorily, but that is not the case; you need to explore why both staff members acted as they did and hear their point of view.

Infection control

Poor infection control practice has risks for patients, staff and the trust and all could have financial as well as personal ramifications. The level of infections within a clinical area is one of the markers for measuring quality control, hence the importance to trusts of education and compliance in this area.

Historically nursing work prior to the 1970s used to be allocated by 'task', with a division of labour, which was first conceived by industrialist Adam Smith in the 1700s, as this was thought to produce the greatest productivity. Individual nurses would carry out single tasks for all the patients in one area. This would reflect their knowledge and seniority and was termed 'task allocation'. For instance, the most junior student would undertake the monitoring of temperature or pulse, or toileting patients, with a more senior one undertaking blood pressure monitoring on all the patients. As the HCA role developed, some of these tasks were delegated to HCAs instead of junior students. The problem is that with this fragmentary approach to care, the holistic needs of the patient are not seen and problems can be missed. Patients were not treated as individuals but as a set of tasks to be carried out; supervision of junior staff was likely to be carried out by the staff one grade higher rather than by qualified nurses or designated mentors. Adam Smith's division of labour in the production of metal nails may have been successful in the short term, but it doesn't work well long-term in industry, and certainly not with sick humans! (For more information on the economic theories that developed from Adam Smith, see Further study.)

There was thus a gradual move to a more coherent workload management – team nursing that provides more continuity of care. In this process both staff and patients were allocated to a team and the teams worked to deliver all the necessary care for those clients, over a number of shifts.

As the teams remained static, staff grew to know their patients better and were able to deliver a more holistic, thorough approach to care. Each team would include both experienced and junior staff and students, so an element of task delegation was also likely to occur, but this was not as pronounced as in task allocation and junior staff were likely to have more direct supervision from qualified staff and mentors. You may have experienced both task and team working on the wards in recent years as there has been some return to these processes, particularly if staffing levels are low.

In the 1980s the concept of primary nursing was brought to the UK from the USA. This workload approach linked each patient to a specific primary nurse, who was an experienced qualified practitioner, and the approach is also called patient allocation. (This should not be confused with primary care, where nursing or medical care takes place in the client's home, rather than in a healthcare setting.) The primary (or named) nurse was responsible for setting and agreeing all nursing care for each client, some of which could be delegated to colleagues. The primary nurse took responsibility for all the care delivered even when not on duty; this proved very difficult to implement effectively in the UK and the practice never became fully established. This way of working was highly people-centred as it gave a large amount of autonomy and thus job satisfaction to the primary nurse; the downside was that it required high levels of trained staff and they were alarmed at being accountable for care delivered in their absence.

The concept of the named nurse did persist for a longer period, when many areas reverted to team nursing, as the team leader was designated as named nurse for all those clients in the team. The objective of the named nurse, from the patient perspective, was to ensure that every patient or client knew at least one nurse who was caring for them. In reality, if the named nurse is only ever the team leader, then this situation fails if the team leader is not on duty. From the nursing perspective the primary nurse (and later the named nurse) role was aimed at improving staff morale, by providing completeness of care for individual clients. To this end it was effective, but the reality of staffing levels in the UK then and since has never really permitted this to occur as intended and there has been a return to a mix of task and team allocation.

If the nursing care of individual clients is fragmented down to individual tasks, there is a risk that, although all activities are completed, the overall well-being of the client is missed. This can lead to loss of quality care and an increase in risk to clients, staff and organisations. In the scenario, team nursing is operating and a specific task, the admission of Mr Jones, has been designated to two staff members of differing grades. The delegation to June and Katy reflects task allocation, with appropriate use of experience and expertise. The team leader believed she had delegated work effectively and appropriately and would thus be making efficient use of her available staff resources, reducing risk and maintaining high-quality care.

Activity 6.4   *Leadership and management*

How is work allocated in your area of practice at the moment?

As this is a personal reflection, no outline answer is supplied.

In the activity you may have identified that work is divided by task, team or named nurse strategies, or maybe it is even less organised. There may be rigid team boundaries and no one delivers care to clients not in their team. If you have patient allocation, is it consistent and reasonable and are there enough staff on duty to undertake this? You may also note that there are different ways of working between day and night shifts. As a manager, you need to be aware of how the system works, and where it could be improved; staff need to work as effectively and efficiently as possible at all times.

Managing change to reduce risk

Scenario

After the lunch break you remind Katy and June about the meeting; you have booked the matron's office for privacy and suggest that you are likely to be finished inside half an hour. At the designated hour Katy meets you outside the office, but June is not there and even though the shift hasn't officially finished, you see June leaving the building with her coat and bag. Once inside the room, Katy bursts into tears and through the sobs apologises for June's behaviour. You feel the best strategy is to go and make some tea, allowing Katy to calm down while you do so. With the tea and tissues in place, you ask Katy to explain what happened and why she is so upset.

It appears that June was not very helpful with Mr Jones's admission at all and that Katy ended up demanding that she get the specimen bottle, and this had resulted in an angry response. Katy promptly apologises for her own behaviour and recognises that she should not have become frustrated and angry, particularly in front of a client. You are about to say that you will need to report the outburst to the ward manager, in case there is a complaint from Mr Jones's family. Katy recognises her accountability in this matter and explains that she felt challenged by both the patient's illness and the lack of support from June, but knows she must do better in future.

Katy then asks whether you knew about June's home situation, as she had heard some gossip at lunch time. Katy relates the comment that June had wanted to move to the new ward and reduce her working hours considerably as her husband is terminally ill with lung cancer. The hospital manager had said that with her experience and all the current changes this would not be possible at the moment; it was full-time employment or nothing. June had remained full-time and moved to your ward where she was clearly preoccupied with her husband's health. Clearly gossip can be a breach of confidentiality and should be acted on very carefully, but if this is true it has implications for the way June is managed.

As a manager it is important that the problem is clarified, explored and ultimately resolved to the benefit of both the staff and the workload. You thus reassure Katy about her behaviour and confirm the correctness of her actions, particularly as you know that being so newly qualified she will be anxious about her own accountability (NMC, 2008b). You decide to reflect on the day's activities and the gossip that has been relayed to you and consider if you acted reasonably and, in particular, where the risks lie.

Risk assessment

Task allocation

You reason that from your experience with GP admissions you were right in allocating a trained nurse and an HCA to undertake the admission; this was well within their remit. You were correct in the assumption that Mr Jones was more poorly than might have been inferred from the phone call. You had assessed the risk and planned for it. You have considered both concern for people and production and have demonstrated team management.

Infection control

The level of infection control risk was acceptable with the strategy you implemented; as both staff members were experienced with trust policies they should have been able to manage the situation safely. There should have been minimal risk to Mr Jones, the staff or other patients. You show appropriate, minimal concern for people and more for production, the authority–obedience management style or task allocation.

People management

Third, you could probably not have anticipated the way June behaved today but you reflect that you may not have managed her well. It is clear that you made lots of assumptions about June, based on your previous encounters with HCAs, who had worked on the ward longer than you. You had not really spoken to her at all, asked what she wanted to do or involved her in the decision-making process. You recognise she represented a considerable risk to the safe function of the unit, and this is an example of impoverished management as you have little concern for people and little for production. This could result in considerable risk to the organisation at all levels. Had you spoken briefly to June at the start of the shift you might have engendered a better rapport with her; or realised that there were underlying problems and that she might not have been able to deal with a difficult emotional situation. However, it is important that workers realise that, unless they discuss their problems with colleagues in a professional manner, it is likely to be assumed that they will function effectively all the time.

Mandatory training has been implemented in all organisations to reduce risks to patients, staff and the organisation and to meet legal requirements. Typically within the health sector, training is provided to *all* staff in topics such as fire prevention, moving and manual handling, health and safety at work, infection control and confidentiality. It would thus be reasonable to expect an established member of staff, such as June, to have a basic understanding of these areas.

Scenario

As Heather, the ward manager, is on duty in the morning, you take the opportunity to ring her at home to set up a brief meeting about June tomorrow. The ward manager says that she has already had a phone call from June informing that she'll be off sick tomorrow, as

continued . . .

she went home unwell. You are taken aback by this and say that she seemed OK at work but that there were problems with her work; you arrange to come in early the following day to meet up.

When you get home later you decide to write down the events in a chronological order as clearly as you can, to allow you to reflect further.

When you and Heather meet, she asks you to describe what happened and you are pleased that your notes make the morning's events follow a logical order, with nothing missed out. Heather says that she feels you did nothing wrong and that your leadership was clear and logical, but that she was at fault by not telling you about June's problems. Heather apologised for not discussing the problems associated with June's appointment to the ward team, as she had not realised that it would cause such immediate problems, and she had tried to maintain June's confidentiality.

As the meeting progresses you ask how Mr Jones is progressing and are informed that his condition has stabilised but the MRSA screen has come back positive. Heather thus congratulates you on your risk assessment skills and your forward planning when placing Mr Jones in a side ward.

MRSA infections have high levels of morbidity and mortality and the prompt implementation of infection control policies as a precaution will have saved the trust from potential additional problems.

Witness statements

Activity 6.5 — *Communication*

Try to write a formal statement about a recent event at work. It doesn't have to be a problem or unusual, just an event you think you can recall.

There is guidance on this activity at the end of the chapter.

Writing witness statements can be difficult and if you have never had to do one before you should seek guidance. Dimond (2011, p211) details when a statement might be required. Some are concerned with criminal proceedings, others with civil or tribunal proceedings and the one concerning a death would be part of a coroner's case. They are statements:

*   to the police concerning a criminal act by a patient or employee;
*   to the police about one's own involvement in a criminal act, but you have the right not to incriminate yourself (the equivalent of remaining silent);
*   to a senior employee about an incident, loss of property, accident, complaint or death;
*   to a senior employee about your conduct or absenteeism;

- to a senior employee about someone else as part of a disciplinary process;
- about an accident to self or colleague.

In criminal cases one is obliged to make a statement and in other situations a good statement acts as a prompt for one's memory, as it may be many months before any meeting takes place.

Dimond (2011, p213) also notes the essentials of a statement, which must be factual, relevant and have clarity. They are:

- date and time of any incident;
- full name of statement maker, position, grade and location;
- full name of any person involved;
- full and detailed description of event;
- signature;
- any supporting statement or documents attached (or equipment kept for examination).

Confidentiality

Confidentiality is an aspect of nursing with which you will be familiar from your pre-registration programme and is discussed at length in the *Code of Conduct* (NMC, 2008b), but you may only have considered it in the context of clients, not in personnel terms. It can be very difficult for managers to know how much information to communicate or disclose with others concerning a member of staff, as there are many areas of legislation (Dimond, 2011).

In the scenario, Heather should have met with June to explain the trust's decision and to talk through any options and the rationale for her appointment on your ward. In particular, as June is under considerable stress, she may have needed a period of compassionate or health-related leave. There is considerable evidence to support the belief that issues at work or healthcare needs of relatives can cause considerable stress and illness (there is more on this in Chapter 8). It would appear from the scenario that no attempt has been made to accommodate June's needs effectively; should June feel that she has no option but to resign from the post, she may well be able to sue for constructive dismissal (Dimond, 2011). Constructive dismissal is when an employee resigns from an organisation because the employee feels that his or her contract has already been breached by the employer. As the employer has not met his or her part of the employment bargain, the contract has been breached by the employer and this equates to dismissal.

Scenario

When June is back from sick leave, Heather sets up a meeting with you all, to enable a frank and open discussion about the incident. She stresses that it is important that, rather than apportion blame, the incident is reviewed and a way forward agreed.

Heather makes the team aware that she is happy to talk about stressful situations be they at home or work, and if she knows of the problem will help manage it effectively. She also

continued . . .

agrees to approach the trust to discuss June's situation more fully and get an outcome satisfactory to June and the trust.

You and Katy are reassured that you did the right thing in terms of the potential MRSA infection, but that you both may need more training in people management, which Heather agrees to look into.

June apologises for the way she behaved and recognises the risks that she created. She also knows that she must talk about the stresses she is under and agrees to seek help through her GP or counselling services.

Managing the risks associated with infections is a high priority for today's health services. MRSA is being managed better in the UK and the incidence of 1,230 deaths due to it in 2008 was down to 485 in 2011; but it is still implicated in a range of problems. Other organisms that have profound implications for healthcare settings are *Clostridium difficile* and norovirus and the means of preventing cross-infection should be understood by all grades of staff.

Hence healthcare organisations need to build infection control information into annual staff mandatory training and updates. Infection control training is vital, so that staff remain aware of how to prevent cross-infection, which is costly to both patients and staff. Much data is collected by in-house teams on the incidence of infection and the duration of outbreaks, so that they can be managed effectively. This material will then be used by the organisation as part of its clinical governance strategy and quality monitoring, as well as submitting the data as part of national epidemiological evidence.

Conclusion

In this chapter, the way that the team leader managed a situation has illustrated management styles that reflect either a person- or a task-centred outlook. Managing the risks associated with any infection must be a high priority for any organisation and high-quality standards have to be maintained. However, it is also vitally important in any organisation to recognise that changes to the workplace can cause stress and when there are also stressors at home, staff may be in an intolerable position.

Activities: brief outline answers

Activity 6.1

You should have recalled the NMC requirements and your local trust/organisational protocols for oral, intravenous or controlled drugs. You need to be familiar with this type of information to explain to students.

Activity 6.2

Emergency situations such as a cardiac arrest or unexpected fit clearly override other work activities and staff will frequently participate for longer than is usual in this case. However you may recall work areas where it was routine for you to work without breaks or go home late. In these situations, managers should consider what is happening and why, so that improvements can be made that are more realistic and less stressful.

Activity 6.3

You should have considered when you should be wearing protective clothing and how to dispose of it correctly. Also think about the way MRSA is screened for and the potential effect of contamination of the clean room environment, if the patient was an MRSA carrier. You may have considered whether a side room is adequate for effective barrier nursing. Work available online from the National Institute for health and Clinical Excellence (NICE) is helpful, at **www.nice.org.uk/guidance/CG2**.

Activity 6.5

Can you remember everything that happened? Even if you can, is it in the right order? Is the time accurate? It is likely that if you write a statement and then read it through you will remember other things. Have you written anything that you 'think happened' or was gossip? Formal statements have to have just the facts, with no 'perhaps' or 'maybe'.

Further reading and useful websites

www.adamsmith.org/adam-smith

Contains more information on the economic theories that developed from Adam Smith.

www.evidence.nhs.uk/search?q=record%20keeping%20Bridget%20Dimond

For articles on nursing and the law, try Bridget Dimond online.

www.internurse.com/cgi-bin/go.pl/library/contents.html?uid=338;journal_uid=9

An online archive of articles including legal issues.

www.nice.org.uk/guidance/

NICE publishes extensively on clinical governance issues.

www.nhs.uk/conditions/

NHS Choices provides up-to-date online information on a variety of topics, including infections.

www.nursingtimes.net/whats-new-in-nursing/news-topics/ethics-and-law-in-nursing/

Nursing Times online has a section on nursing ethics and the law.

Chapter 7
Nursing the deteriorating patient

> ### Chapter aims
>
> After reading this chapter, you will be able to:
>
> - communicate information about patient deterioration;
> - show how team work and clinical decision-making affect care.

Introduction

As a student nurse you will have been used to having your mentor confirm what you do in practice as correct, and even though you will have been exposed to a considerable amount of information on accountability, it may not have felt real. Now as a qualified nurse you are responsible and accountable for your actions to the patient, your employing organisation and the profession at all times (NMC, 2008b). In this chapter there will be some clinical material, notably a brief overview about recognising the deteriorating patient, but it really focuses on the decisions that you need to make in managing any situation and the way that you communicate with others in the patient's interests.

As a student you may have felt awkward asking questions of some of your mentors; perhaps they always seemed too busy or brushed you aside. As a trained staff member you may now feel that you should have the knowledge, that your pre-registration education should have given you all the answers – it will not have done so. Nurse education up to registration only really prepares you for a generic, unspecific role, albeit with lots of regulations and the potential for litigation. To me the first years as a staff nurse are those in which you really learn your craft; you focus your attention on particular types of patient care and you grow in knowledge, skills and attitudes. You must now actively seek out answers to questions; you mustn't be embarrassed by what you don't know. The important thing is to know what it is you don't know, and to find answers. I believe that if you express a reasonable interest in a topic, most medical, nursing or allied health profession staff will be willing to share their knowledge with you; after all, patients may well be asking similar questions. Lifelong learning means just that: you will always be seeking out new knowledge, skills or attitudes wherever they may be found; never lose your thirst for learning.

Interprofessional working

> ### Scenario
>
> You are a newly appointed staff nurse in a day-case theatre unit at a private hospital, which is a practice area you spent time on during your training, at the start of the second year. You were pleased to be offered this post, which is part of a rotational scheme within the whole theatre suite. You are expected to spend three months in this unit before moving for

continued . . .

a further three months in each of the following: main theatres, the recovery department and the endoscopy unit. While on the rotation scheme you are undertaking a formalised preceptorship programme, which is offered to all newly qualified staff from all disciplines in the organisation. The interdisciplinary nature of the preceptorshp programme has been really interesting, as the sharing of experiences and the realities of responsibility and accountability are being discussed at length and with great feeling. The programme has also included some shared clinical role-play situations and this has really helped clarify roles and responsibilities in emergency-type situations; this is particularly relevant as your hospital has no intensive care unit.

Today you are working in the recovery room on the day-case unit, which cares for patients having a wide range of both adult and child surgical procedures. The unit has a policy of carefully screening all patients prior to day surgery, to ensure that they are fit and well and should be able to return home after any procedure. In this way it is hoped that patients will follow a routine plan of care and that emergency problems will very rarely occur.

Today the surgeons in theatre are carrying out an orthopaedic list, which includes knee and other joint arthroscopic procedures and removal of bunions. Ms Jones was seen in the outpatient department (OPD) one month ago, following a referral from her GP. She has bunions on both feet and these are not only restricting her footwear but giving her pain, where they rub. At the OPD visit Ms Jones was noted to be fit and well, with no apparent health issues other than her bilateral bunions. She had been a smoker but had given up several years ago and was not overweight, so she was expected to make a full recovery from the surgery, following the anticipated care pathway.

Much of this chapter deals with interprofessional working, so the first activity is a reflection on your own experiences.

Activity 7.1   *Reflection*

Take time to consider how interprofessional working is effectively achieved in your clinical area.

An outline answer is provided at the end of the chapter.

Preceptorship programmes have been set up as an adjunct to the current pre-registration programme and reflect how trusts and organisations want to build up the confidence of newly qualified staff. They may allow newly qualified staff to be supernumerary for a period of time or remove them from the clinical area for study days. In these study days, time could be spent exploring clinical situations and reflecting on experiences with the other professionals involved in patient scenarios. They may include a session on recognising and acting for the deteriorating patient or discussing hospital protocols and guidelines, such as integrated care pathways (ICPs).

However, as financial constraints tighten, it may be that this type of supportive programme ceases.

Integrated care pathways

ICPs (British Association of Day Surgery, 2004) have been developed as a way of planning the treatment and care for patients having the same routine treatment, the rationale being that most aspects of each patient's treatment will be identical. An agreed ICP will reduce variance in procedure, be evidence-based, reflect both patient experience and clinical judgment and should demonstrate best practice and thus reduce risk. As it is used by all professions involved in the patient's care it should improve communication and enhance safety. In the NHS it will also fit with the electronic patient record system; however, the ICP is a guide rather than a dictate, so can vary if necessary.

Activity 7.2   *Communication*

Do ICPs exist where you work? How are they evaluated, and how do they fit with the clinical governance agenda?

There is guidance on this activity at the end of the chapter.

Clinical governance

Clinical governance arose from the business community with the aim of considering corporate risk, in terms of finances, legal requirements and effective operations (the 'Cadbury code', cited by McSherry and Pearce, 2002). In 1999 the NHS Executive proposed corporate governance in the NHS covering accountability, probity (honesty) and openness (Department of Health, 1999). This was converted into clinical governance, to focus on patient need, best standards and collaborative working and to enhance public confidence in the NHS.

McSherry and Pearce (2002) summarise the clinical governance components as safety, organisational culture, quality improvement/maintenance and professional/organisational accountability.

Clinical governance requires the NHS to continue to improve its service through:

- clinical risk management;
- clinical audit;
- continuing practice and professional development;
- research and development.

The aim, therefore, is to ensure that all the services and care that the NHS delivers are of the highest quality, make best use of the financial resources and meet the needs of the clients and users. To this end local departments such as clinical audit and complaints have developed alongside national institutions such as the National Institute for Health and Clinical Excellence (NICE).

In this scenario, the patient is referred to the surgeon with the diagnosis of bunions by her GP and will have a metatarsal osteotomy on her right foot, which is the more painful foot. In the OPD an assessment will be made, not just of her surgical needs, but also her general well-being and social situation. This is to ensure that she is as fit as possible to undergo a general anaesthetic and to recover safely from it and the surgery. She will then return home later in the day to recover more fully. The first part of the care pathway will include screening for cardiac and lung function and routine blood tests. Ms Jones will also be screened for any existing infections and informed that if she develops a cold or upper respiratory tract infection, surgery will be postponed. The care pathway will also indicate what preoperation preparation is required and how long she should be nil by mouth prior to the surgery. It will also include details of the expected surgical procedure, postoperation recovery and wound dressings, which will be discussed with the patient.

Team work

Scenario

Ms Jones has been told at the OPD appointment that she should have nothing to eat for the six hours prior to surgery and only sips of water after this, ceasing two hours presurgery. This will reduce the risk amount of stomach content and prevent vomiting or gastric reflux in surgery (Creed and Spiers, 2010). Ms Jones is a successful business woman and exudes confidence; she has not expressed any concerns about the surgery either in the OPD or on admission to the day surgery unit. It is not until she is in the anaesthetic room that she admits to being very scared of the potential pain and this is why she opted for a general anaesthetic as opposed to local anaesthesia for the operation.

The surgery goes well and Ms Jones arrives into the recovery room. Her airway is protected by a laryngeal mask (Anaesthesia UK, 2010) and the anaesthetist, concerned about her pain levels, has just administered 5mg IV morphine, which is within safe limits but a relatively high dose.

Using an ABCDE structured approach, you carry out a rapid assessment of Ms Jones's needs.

ABCDE structured assessment

There has been considerable concern within the health service, culminating in a report from the Department of Health in 2000, about the need to recognise and act on the deteriorating patient more quickly (Department of Health, 2000a). The use of a structured tool such as ABCDE with a 'look, listen and feel' approach (Creed and Spiers, 2010) should mean that a worsening patient situation is recognised quickly. However, this is not always the case and recording the assessments on a chart should contribute to a 'track and trigger' system. This score will then alert staff to act quickly due to a combination of physiological changes. In your training you will have covered basic life support and some first aid and may have spent time working with acutely ill patients in intensive care units, theatres or the emergency room (but you might not), or your skills might be rusty. This quick refresher should also prompt you to discuss ABCDE and assessment when you are mentoring a student or healthcare assistant (HCA). It is also worth trying to access a short course such as the ALERT programme in your trust. This course and others like it help you recognise and act quickly as patients deteriorate (Smith, 2003, cited by Creed and Spiers, 2010).

Theory summary: ABCDE

- Airway: look for signs of obstruction to the airway. If there is complete obstruction there will be silence, but partial obstruction to the airway may be accompanied by abnormal sounds such as a wheeze or stridor. Note the situation of any airway adjuncts also.
- Breathing: look, listen and feel for rate and depth of breathing; consider the breathing pattern and whether the accessory muscles are used. In addition, listening to chest sounds and recording the oxygen saturations can be helpful; it should also be noted if the patient has oxygen administered. Oxygen saturation levels (PaO_2) will reflect both breathing and circulation.
- Circulation: again, look, listen and feel. Monitoring the pulse, note its rate, rhythm and strength, as well as blood pressure, colour and temperature of skin and capillary refill time.
- Disability: this is a broader area and may encompass a neurological assessment such as AVPU (alert, responds to voice, responds to pain, unresponsive) for level of consciousness or the more detailed Glasgow Coma Scale for the unconscious or head-injured patient. It may also encompass blood glucose monitoring, which should be considered in any patient rather than just those known to have diabetes mellitus.
- Exposure: this is a more widespread assessment and, if body temperature hasn't been noted yet, it must be now, as well as looking for sites of injury or pain and swelling. The patient or relatives may be able to give a history of the patient's condition and charts may reveal medication or fluid intake or ECG recording. When exposing the patient for this part of the assessment, care should be taken with dignity, privacy and to prevent loss of warmth.

It may be that you are providing one-to-one care, as in the scenario, and need to recognise changes and act quickly. Unfortunately, despite the correct use of the structured ABCDE assessment, it was noted that staff did not recognise the significance of changes in the patient's status until they had deteriorated severely. Hence the development of 'track and trigger' systems (NICE, 2007), which prompt the practitioner, when certain criteria are encountered, to take swift action. All acute care trusts were recommended to implement this system, but there are slightly varying parameters and a variety of names, such as Early Warning System (EWS) or Modified Early Warning System (MEWS) or Patient at Risk Score (PARS). Trusts have also frequently incorporated the system within routine observation paperwork for acutely ill patients.

Activity 7.3   *Leadership and management*

What 'track and trigger' system is used where you work? Is it incorporated in routine paperwork? This activity should prompt you to seek out the resources of your own organisation and perhaps enrol on a programme.

As this is an individual activity, no outline answer is given.

It is apparent that, in many situations, a patient's respiratory (breathing) rate is no longer being routinely monitored and this may be due to the use of electronic equipment to record pulse rate, pulse oximetry and blood pressure. Unfortunately, the equipment cannot judge the breathing rate, nor assess the strength of a pulse or the clamminess of the skin, so these are not commented on. This is why some organisations have returned to manual monitoring systems for blood pressure and pulse and staff have to relearn traditional nursing skills such as discreetly counting respiratory rate.

Change in the respiratory rate is one of the earliest and most significant changes in the deteriorating patient and happens due to a variety of causes (Creed and Spiers, 2010). An increase in respiratory rate may indicate a need to increase oxygen intake or remove carbon dioxide; it is linked to regulation of the acid–base balance (pH) and to changes in the central nervous system. It is stated that a respiratory rate of less than ten, or more than 24, breaths per minute in an adult may well be a cause for concern, particularly when there are other signs of physiological instability.

Changes in pulse rate and rhythm are also significant in an adult. Less than 60 beats per minute or more than 100 may be of concern; changes in pulse rate may appear later than changes in respiratory rate. Tachycardia is a compensatory mechanism in acute illness and is an attempt by the body to increase cardiac output.

Changes in blood pressure occur late in acute illness and it is usual to find the trigger for an 'alert' on an early-warning score when the systolic blood pressure falls below 100mmHg. A mean arterial pressure of less than 60mmHg is a more reliable indicator of failing tissue perfusion (Creed and Spiers, 2010).

Other observations that may well be significant are the PaO_2 reading, the level of consciousness and body temperature, coupled with fluid balance, level of pain and changes in blood analysis, but in all these readings it is the small changes that are as significant as the overall reading.

Overall changes in respiratory rate, pulse and blood pressure are indicators of the development of shock, which may not be reversible. With the use of documentation that captures 'track and trigger' cues, it is hoped that the deterioration of a patient can be identified quickly and acted on effectively.

Activity 7.4   *Reflection*

Are you quite sure that all staff to whom you delegate the observation of vital signs understand the significance of what they are doing, and why accuracy is important?

As this is a personal reflection, no outline answer is supplied.

You must remember that when you delegate tasks to untrained staff, you remain accountable for their actions. So you must be confident in their capability to undertake a task and to report back findings appropriately.

Aspects of the scenario should have parallels in your own work situation. For instance, are you fully familiar with all the equipment that is available to support patient care and how it works?

Activity 7.5   *Critical thinking*

If a student approached you to ask the reason why the following tasks are performed, what would your comprehensive, knowledgeable answer be?

1. Why do staff check the light bulb works on a laryngoscope?
2. Why should I learn to feel for a manual radial pulse, when the electronic monitoring equipment is quicker?
3. Why do you appear to be taking the pulse and then documenting the breathing rate?

An outline answer is provided at the end of the chapter.

Good communication

Scenario

Ms Jones remains unconscious when she is wheeled from the theatre suite into the recovery area, which is rather unusual, as you have noticed that many patients are often awakening; sometimes you even wonder if they have actually been unconscious during surgery. You rapidly undertake an ABCDE assessment and note that her airway is protected by the laryngeal mask airway (LMA) in situ, but that her breathing rate is slow, at only eight breaths per minute. You attach an electronic monitoring system which records blood pressure, pulse and pulse oximetry to monitor circulation and all are within normal parameters, and you jot down the time Ms Jones came to you. You stay with your patient, closely monitoring her and plan to record the vital signs every 15 minutes. As Ms Jones was the last client on the surgery list, the anaesthetist looks into the recovery unit, asks if everything is all right and before you have really gathered your thoughts, he has dis-

---

continued . . .

appeared. The orthopaedic surgeon who carried out the surgery has already said goodbye and said that he would see Ms Jones as an outpatient; her follow-up care is written in her notes.

Ms Jones seems to be about to wake up but also starts to become restless, suggesting to you that she is in pain. You would like to remove the LMA in case it is causing her distress, but even though her blood pressure and pulse are satisfactory, her respiratory rate is still only ten breaths per minute and she hasn't really exhibited signs that she might be able to protect her own airway. She doesn't yet respond to your voice. You are concerned about the patient's pain level but also aware that if she has more opiate analgesic she may depress her respiratory rate further. You decide to seek help.

It should have been apparent that the potential problem in this scenario is the slow respiratory rate, that would be a cause for some concern on a 'track and trigger' scheme, although the oxygen saturations (PaO_2) may well be satisfactory. The risk is the need to reduce the patient's level of pain without further slowing the respiratory rate and also ensure that she is fit for discharge home.

Having recognised the potential risk of harm to the patient and your own inexperience, you decide to instigate some type of effective action.

The SPAR communication tool

Communicating effectively with colleagues is a key aspect of effective healthcare, and one of the tools recommended to help do this effectively is SBAR (situation, background, assessment, recommendations). Using this tool should ensure that the caller makes the responder understand the seriousness of the situation, where the problem exists and what the responder is expected to do.

Situation

The caller states where he or she and the casualty/patient are situated; this enables the responder to arrive at the correct destination. For instance, in the scenario, the patient is in the recovery area attached to the day-case unit. A member of the medical staff receiving your call may assume that recovery is attached to the main theatre suite and therefore go to the wrong place. The situation also allows you to explain what the problem is; in this scenario the patient has a slow respiratory rate and is not yet fully conscious, yet appears to be in pain.

Background

The background information allows an explanation of what has already happened. In this case, that would be the type of surgery performed, the slow return to consciousness, the observation of vital signs, in particular the respiratory rate, and the analgesia already given.

Assessment

At this point the problem or potential problem is explained. Ms Jones requires more analgesia, but the only one prescribed is an intravenous opiate and her somewhat depressed respiratory rate might be worsened by more opiates. Ms Jones is a day-case patient due to go home in four hours.

Recommendations

This is what the caller wants to happen and in this situation a return visit from the anaesthetist might be the foremost requirement. If this is not possible, then the caller wants patient assessment by a more experienced staff member.

SBAR has been developed because communication in critical situations has been found to be poor, because as people become anxious they frequently become less organised. When the sender uses SBAR, each phase of the message is included and the recipient is provided with a realistic picture of the problem and what is required.

In this scenario it is clear that the Ms Jones' condition needs to be considered by a more experienced member of staff quickly. As her respiratory rate is low, additional opiate analgesia may have a detrimental effect depressing it further, even though her PaO_2 reading may currently be satisfactory. However, without effective analgesia she is unlikely to feel able to go home later. The Department of Health (2009) identifies a chain of response for the deteriorating patient, so that junior staff are provided with access to more senior and knowledgeable support as required (Figure 7.1).

Recorder → Recogniser → Primary responder → Secondary responder → Tertiary responder (critical care).

Figure 7.1. Chain of response for the deteriorating patient (adapted from Creed and Spiers, 2010).

In this scenario, as the staff nurse in recovery you are both recorder and recogniser of a problem, and it may be that your primary responder is a more senior nurse or operating department practitioner. The secondary responder would be the anaesthetist; the tertiary response would be movement from the day-case area to an inpatient ward or, if the situation warranted it, to the local critical care facility.

Scenario

You bleep the day-surgery manager (the first responder), who comes to assess your patient. As the PaO_2 readings remain satisfactory and the LMA is still in situ and is not yet causing Ms Jones distress, he advises a watch-and-wait strategy, checking again in five minutes. He also suggests ringing the anaesthetist as he will still be in the hospital; which you do, explaining the situation again, using the SBAR framework. He acknowledges that he had

continued . . .

prescribed a relatively large intravenous dose of morphine, as Ms Jones had explained to him about her fear of pain when she was waiting to be anaesthetised. By the time the anaesthetist (the second responder) arrives ten minutes later, Ms Jones has woken up and subsequently indicated that the LMA should be removed. As you have spoken to her, reassuring her of the success of the surgery, she has become calmer and appears to be in less pain. The anaesthetist reassures you when he reviews the patient, and feels that, once completely alert, her respiratory rate and pain levels will all be within acceptable parameters.

Activity 7.6   *Decision-making*

Identify three or four possible problems which could have prevented the chain or response being effective in the scenario.

Whatever setting you are working in, you should familiarise yourself with this chain of response and know who would be your primary, secondary and tertiary responders.

An outline answer is provided at the end of the chapter.

Communication is a very important aspect of management and leadership. It is not just in critical situations that it can go wrong, so this chapter will now consider some other ways of improving it. I imagine that when you started your nursing programme you spent considerable time on verbal and non-verbal communication and thought that this was just common sense. If this is so, why is government in 2012 concerned that nurses need to talk to their patients more (*Nursing Standard*, 2012)?

Effective communication is a means of preventing patient/client concerns being missed and tragedies occurring. Goodman and Clemow (2008) write at length about incidences where poor communication, and hence poor collaborative practice, led to the deaths of children, Victoria Climbie in 2000 being only one of a number. In other arenas, such as the Bristol Royal Infirmary inquiry, and in the case of Harold Shipman, opportunities were missed to communicate and act on reported untoward occurrences. It is thus a recognised fact that the quality of healthcare depends as much on the communication between employees and employers and outside bodies as it does on what actually takes place. In a system run by people, things will go wrong; the important thing is to have systems in place to spot these problems early.

Wilkinson (1997, cited by Kelemen, 2003) identifies the need to educate workers in the recognition of organisational issues, allow them to take control of their working environment and, importantly, managers must listen to their view on problem-solving. This translates into a bottom-up approach to improving quality. Nurses talking directly and frequently to patients is most definitely a bottom-up approach to patient care.

But talking to patients will not effect change unless the patient's voice is listened to and acted on. Similarly, check sheets and tick boxes are designed as proof of tasks carried out, not as prompts, and should not use more time and effort than is actually available. Qualified nurses should observe the activity of students and HCAs much more thoroughly, supporting and guiding them. In this way correct communication, care and attitudes to patients are learnt.

Poor communication between members of a team may reflect a whole range of problems and in the current health service an apparent lack of a common language may be one of them. A registered nurse within the EU has a right to work in the UK, and be registered with the NMC, which does not assess language levels. This is an issue for the employing authority (NMC, 2007). A multicultural society has many benefits but it can have a downside, not least in regard to language, interpretation and role expectations. Women and nurses in some cultures may still be perceived as secondary to men and doctors, yet if communication in a team is to be effective, all participants must be able to express their views equally.

Methods of communication

Powell and Brodsky (1998), writing about clinical supervision, note that in any message via whatever route there are many stages. Firstly, there must be a sender with thoughts and emotions. Then there is the message itself, with its content and its channel of communication; there will also be 'noise' – the way a message may be disrupted. Finally there is reception, and feedback.

Powell also cites Watzlawick et al. (1967), who suggest that *we can't not communicate*, insofar as every message, or lack of it, means something. Also, by sending a message, or not sending one to an individual, we make assumptions about that person. For instance, does the old adage 'no news is good news' still apply when there are so many means of electronic communication?

In a similar vein, not sending a message cannot be seen in isolation but as part of a set of messages that reflect the relationship of the sender and receiver. For instance, you might say to your partner before leaving for a night out that you won't ring unless there is a problem getting a taxi home. The unspoken message is: 'don't wait up'.

Putting this into the context of the scenario, if you don't ask for help with Ms Jones, there is an assumption that you are able to manage the situation. In contrast, if you use SBAR to contact a primary responder to deal with Ms Jones' potential problems, you are illustrating your concerns in a professional and competent way. A logical, clearly communicated concern with a specific request for action is unlikely to be misinterpreted; furthermore any subsequent action can also be explained.

Thinking back to those communication exercises that took place in your pre-registration programme will, I am sure, conjure up terms like verbal and non-verbal communication or personal space. It is important to remember that, although you probably learnt about these in terms of staff–patient/client interactions, there is also much to consider in staff interactions.

For instance, you may be aware of bodily contact or personal space when carrying out intimate care or providing comfort, but what about when you have to hold a disciplinary-type meeting? How do you show empathy but not shy away from dealing with a problem? What about body posture or the position of the table and chairs in a meeting, do you want to be the 'chair' in a position of power or 'one of the boys'? These are the communication issues of leadership, and although apparently trivial, can have considerable implications, particularly when a patient's well-being may be in the balance.

Bach and Ellis (2011) write about team work and how effectiveness is improved by shared goals, a willingness to discuss and listen, to give and receive feedback and handle disagreements positively and openly – in other words, to have effective communication. They also refer to the work of Sullivan and Decker (2009), who feel that organisational roles will affect communication; some staff are task-focused and thus use discussions, opinions, documentation and all manner of communication to get the task completed. Others take a nurturing role, and will be concerned with the way individuals interact and on interpersonal needs. In reality a manager may take a different role depending on the situation and in large organisations the employees may themselves have different roles. Ultimately the way leaders, managers and staff work together will affect not only the tasks to be achieved and the patient care but also the morale and success of the team.

Belbin, as early as the 1970s, was working on the roles individuals play within teams and showed how an effective balance of the roles gets the activities completed most successfully. Belbin identified nine role types in any organisation and that each individual type of team role has both a positive and negative side to the character. Having too many of the same type of characteristic can be unhelpful and even destructive. As a piece of useful research, explore Belbin's work (see Further study).

Activities: brief outline answers

Activity 7.1

You might have identified multidisciplinary team meetings, or case conferences or you might consider that the nursing staff act as a relay for the other professionals, who work independently of each other. Either way, do you find that care is seamlessly transferred between professional groups or does it occasionally fail?

Activity 7.2

If your trust or organisation does not subscribe to ICP you should consider looking at ICPs available online to suit your care area. The introduction of ICPs could be used as a topic for discussion in a clinical meeting with your colleagues. Alternatively you may have considered the work of the clinical governance department in your trust, and how it impinges on the care you deliver.

Activity 7.5

This is really about making sure you are up to speed with all the resuscitation equipment in your area. You should be able to say that even in an emergency you could identify and work all the required equipment quickly. You should also be able to reassure yourself that it is always clean and fully functioning and discuss its use with a junior colleague.

1. A laryngoscope is an illuminated tool used by the anaesthetist to depress the tongue and then inspect the airway as far as the vocal cords. This is frequently used at the start of intubation and may be needed rapidly in an emergency situation.
2. Taking a radial pulse manually for one minute allows you to consider not only the rate, but also the rhythm and strength of the beats, which an electronic system cannot.

3. It is important to count breathing rate when the patient is not aware of this happening, as everyone tends to alter their breathing rate when they are made aware of it. Hence staff frequently take the 'pulse' for longer than necessary as they are actually counting the breathing rate.

Activity 7.6

In the scenario, you might not have recorded the low respiratory rate of the patient. You might not have responded to these signs. The anaesthetist might have already left the building, and be out of communication. Other more senior staff might have been unavailable, non-responding or dealing with emergencies.

You should know how to contact help in case an emergency arises; knowing what you should have done, after an emergency, will be of no consolation. This is particularly important information to communicate to junior colleagues if you work outside a district general hospital, as it may be that phoning 999 for paramedic support is the only option.

Further reading and useful websites

Belbin's work and resources can be found at **www.belbin.com**

www.clinicalgovernance.scot.nhs.uk/section2/pathways.asp

www.medicine.ox.ac.uk/bandolier/booth/glossary/icp.html

These sites are good sources of information on ICPs.

www.expressyourselftosuccess.com/three-benefits-of-improving-communication-skills/

www.helpguide.org/mental/effective_communication_skills.htm

Both these sites are good on improving communication at work or in relationships.

www.patientsafetyfirst.nhs.uk/Content.aspx?path=/interventions/Criticalcare/

More information on recognising the deteriorating patient.

www.rcn.org.uk/__data/assets/pdf_file/0003/381099/2011_RCN_research_S15.pdf

Read the comprehensive RCN report online recognising the deteriorating patient.

Chapter 8
How to manage competing demands

NMC Standards for Pre-registration Nursing Education

This chapter will address the following competencies:

Domain 2: Communication and interpersonal skills

1. All nurses must build on partnerships and therapeutic relationships through safe, effective and non-discriminatory communication. They must take account of individual differences, capabilities and needs.

Domain 3: Nursing practice and decision-making

1. All nurses must . . . make person-centred, evidence-based judgements and decisions, in partnership with others involved in the care process, to ensure high quality care . . .

NMC Essential Skills Clusters

This chapter will address the following ESCs:

Cluster: Care, compassion and communication

1. As partners in the care process, people can trust a newly registered graduate nurse to provide collaborative care based on the highest standards, knowledge and competence.

By entry to register

12. Recognises and acts to overcome barriers in developing effective relationships with service users and carers.

Cluster: Organisational aspects of care

9. People can trust the newly registered graduate nurse to treat them as partners and work with them to make a holistic and systematic assessment of their needs; to develop a personalised plan that is based on mutual understanding and respect for their individual situation promoting health and well-being, minimising risk of harm and promoting their safety at all times.

By entry to register

13. Acts autonomously and takes responsibility for collaborative assessment and planning of care delivery with the person, their carer and their family.

Chapter aims

After reading this chapter, you will be able to:

- understand how to manage your own workload;
- deal with competing pressures;
- prioritise competing demands for care for patients.

Introduction

The scenarios in this chapter are in both the acute and community settings, and consider the issues of patient dependence and the prioritising of workload. We will focus on decision-making, quality of care and maintaining standards, and will discuss the role of the clinical audit and local governance as well as working with colleagues.

Managing your workload

Competing demands affect us all, and not all of them revolve around work. Sometimes it is possible to sympathise with someone else's demanding life schedule and not see that one's own is as difficult. Educationalists encounter every possible demand placed on a student and sometimes marvel at how they cope and wonder why others have made life so difficult! The workload and competing pressures experienced by the nursing or midwifery student are frequently underestimated by students in their first year, or by their family. As you have been through all the assorted traumas that the pre-registration programme has thrown at you, you may well feel that life should get easier now. Don't bank on it. The accountability will weigh heavier and the responsibility you will feel to your 'forever' working colleagues will grow large. Your partner or family may now feel that it is time for them, as they have supported you over three years. They believe that now you must give up things for them, just when you need to develop your own confidence and skills, without a mentor. Perhaps you have moved to a new locality for a job or have been obliged to settle for a post that you feel is less than ideal; those feelings of relief when you completed the programme and awaited your NMC PIN number may be long forgotten. So now you must start reviewing your new 'qualified' life and how best to manage it; this will be about reviewing how you work and also about reviewing the organisation you work in.

The first part of the chapter will be about you and your style of working and later we will consider how teams can best function to maintain high-quality care.

Scenario

Towards the end of your pre-registration programme, your partner, who has always seemed very supportive of your studies, applied for and obtained promotion in another part of the country. You agreed that if he liked the job, you would move home and relocate to be with him; of course this means finding work in a new trust. He has also indicated that perhaps you can start a family, something you'd also eventually like, but can't see in the immediate future. Neither of you have friends or family in this part of the country; on the day you leave your old trust and home, you find yourself in floods of tears.

Fortunately you have been successful in getting a part-time post in the district general hospital midwifery unit, although it is fewer hours than you would have liked and contains a rotation to night duty every six weeks. On a positive note, the unit manager has explained that you will work in all areas and so maintain your skills. You rationalise that working two long shifts a week rather than three might allow you to get to know the locality better, but your partner is concerned about the reduced income and clearing your student debt. In fact you are surprised at how negative he is about the post, even though you explain that knowing the trust may help you identify further opportunities more easily.

Activity 8.1   *Reflection*

Did you leave home to undertake your pre-registration programme? What were the major stressors outside the course work?

As this is an individual activity, no outline answer is provided.

You may have reflected on what caused you most stress as a student and are now clear that all of these stressors have been removed – or perhaps they haven't. If the stressors are still in place, even though you are no longer studying full-time, perhaps you need to look deeper at your lifestyle.

Leaving your 'comfort zone' can be a very stressful situation and research on life stressors has indicated that, other than bereavement and divorce, moving house and changing jobs are incredibly demanding. Even activities that we would consider positive can have a high stress factor: getting married, for instance, scores 50/100 and the tragic death of a spouse is rated 100/100 (see end of chapter for online resources). So it is really important to recognise that, however much you try to be calm and work through problems, stress can have a detrimental effect because of the accumulation of 'points' rather than one major life-changing event.

Dealing with competing pressures

Scenario

It is day one on the unit, and you, like most of the other staff, work long days, which in your case means two shifts a week, today and tomorrow. The unit is very busy, but the manager has indicated that you should work with the same experienced member of the team, to orient yourself, for both days. This seems a very fair start to the job and you are even more pleased when the manager says she wants to meet up and evaluate your experiences at the end of tomorrow's shift. Most staff are friendly and welcoming, but your mentor seems less than pleased to have to 'watch over you', as she puts it. You reassure her that you do have a little postqualifying midwifery experience, although you are not familiar with this trust's policies and procedures, so you hope you won't be too much of a burden.

As the shift moves on, the ward clerk informs you that your access to the trust intranet has been approved and that you will be able to log on and access policies for yourself as well as client information. This will be useful as the unit manager has indicated that you should work through the trust's online induction package, as well as having attended the formal induction day last week. The ward clerk is cheerful and chats briefly, asking you where you used to work and hopes you are getting on OK with Deirdre, your mentor. Other staff are equally welcoming and, to your surprise, are also concerned about you working alongside Deirdre, who has been rather distant all morning. Before you go to break you ensure that a colleague has taken over care of your mothers-to-be and that Deirdre knows what is happening; you leave an apparently calm situation for your break. You know that not everyone will take a break, but feel that time out should be encouraged in all but emergency situations. Deirdre is heard to mutter about lack of time for her break as you leave the ward.

Activity 8.3   *Team working*

Why do some staff not take the appropriate rest breaks during a shift? What do you think are the potential problems of staff working through their allocated breaks?

An outline answer is provided at the end of the chapter.

The interpretation of the European Working Time Directive (NHS Executive, 1998) indicates the importance of rest in the working week and a good working environment will comply with this for all staff. As a manager you should encourage staff to take rest breaks and manage this like any other resource in a timely and effective manner. Staff are the most costly resource an organisation has, and yet managers frequently treat staff less carefully than they would a piece of machinery. However, some staff seem to feel they are indispensable and can't be replaced, even temporarily.

Scenario

As you return to your clients and thank your colleague for her assistance, you notice that Deirdre has still apparently not left her work area, so you ask if you can be of any help, in particular whether someone can take over for a while. Deirdre's response is quite abrupt and clearly indicates that she is far too busy to leave, but it appears that her clients are all stable. You notice that the area for which Deirdre is responsible is quite untidy and Deirdre appears to have a pile of paperwork around her. Still the shift progresses, Deirdre responds reasonably to your occasional query about local policy and the clients are comfortable. Later you take time to make a cup of tea for yourself and Deirdre, as this is permitted on the ward, but you notice she lets it go cold before taking a swift gulp; she is looking harassed and tired. Towards the end of the day, the night staff come on duty and you prepare to hand over your clients, feeling generally pleased with how the day has gone. Unfortunately, Deirdre still appears burdened with paperwork and you wonder what you have forgotten to do. At the bedside handover you cross-examine the incoming midwife for anything that you should have done, but he reassures you all seems fine and you go home.

At home your partner is pleased to see you, but you note that, despite a request, he hasn't considered what meal to prepare. You wonder how your partner would have felt on his first day if expected to plan the evening meal.

The following day, you arrive at work to find that Deirdre is off sick and comments such as 'typical' are being bandied around. You meet the staff who have been on duty overnight and get up to speed with your clients. The ward manager is working clinically today, in Deirdre's absence, and during the morning she asks you about your shift yesterday.

Time management

It would seem from the scenario that Deirdre may not be able to manage her time well and thus she gets over-tired and stressed. Time management is a key aspect of effective working practice and anyone who fails to meet deadlines regularly should consider their working practices. If you consider some situations, the Pareto principle (La Monica Rigolosi, 2005, citing Vilfredo Pareto) would seem to apply, when only 20% of the time is spent on achieving 80% of vital tasks. Alternatively 80% of the time is spent on the tasks that bring in only 20% of the rewards! Although you may not be able to quantify your position to 20:80, are there times when you put off doing vital tasks to concentrate on trivia? Do the cupboards at home suddenly need cleaning when you should be writing an essay or do you watch an interesting programme on TV when you should be cooking tea?

If you know that you don't use your time well, and this may well be the situation with Deirdre in the scenario, you need to spend a little of this valuable commodity trying to improve. You should ask yourself honestly if you are bad at managing your time both at home and at work; if you do then this is likely to cause stress.

Activity 8.4   *Reflection*

If you were to break down each day into half-hour slots, what would the day look like? Are any time slots filled with activity (or inactivity) which you could organise better?

An outline answer is provided at the end of the chapter.

In the workplace, people who manage their time well will often avoid interruptions and their methods can be as diverse as:

* making sure that the drug trolley is stocked before starting the round;
* making sure you have prepared the patient and have all the equipment before starting an aseptic technique;
* putting a 'do not disturb' notice on an office door, or going elsewhere to finish an important task or confidential meeting;
* not answering e-mails and texts all day, but having a set time when you are prepared to answer them and having drop-in chat sessions, rather than at any time in the day;
* having a 'to do' list that actually gets done, in priority order or a shopping list that means nothing is forgotten.

Time management is about competing demands, between those you want to do and those you would rather put off until later. Unfortunately in the workplace there is a real need to prioritise appropriately, so that the most important tasks are completed first. One of the difficulties many staff face is deciding how and when to carry out the paperwork associated with nursing or midwifery. It may sometimes appear that the documentation is more important than the care it represents, which is of course incorrect. Part of this stems from concerns about accountability and clinical governance, which emphasise the documentary evidence. Time is taken away from the activities, to provide documentary proof that they have been carried out.

Activity 8.5

Where do you sit when writing up care notes? Is it at the bedside or away from the client?

What are the advantages and disadvantages of these alternatives?

An outline answer is provided at the end of the chapter.

In the scenario, Deirdre appears to be disorganised and unable to manage her time well, as there doesn't appear to be client-oriented emergency that would delay her. So perhaps she is not working as efficiently as she might and hence the burden of having to provide mentoring to a newly appointed member of staff is too much and she goes off sick. Sickness and absenteeism in the workplace are frequently indicators of a poor working environment, particularly if they affect all the staff (European Foundation, 1997).

Consider how it might have been if Deirdre had a different approach to her workload. First, she is delighted to have a new member of staff on the team. She would have engaged you in a brief conversation about orientation to the unit, as it was your first day, and then asked about your postqualifying experience. As a mentor, she would have introduced you to other members of staff as appropriate and perhaps indicated a good time for your break so you could meet other midwifery staff and other key individuals, such as the ward clerk. She might feel that covering your workload for the break is more important than going for break at the same time as you, as this allows you to meet other staff, or she might feel you need a 'friendly face' in the canteen. During the shift as an effective mentor to a qualified midwife, Deirdre would ask how things were progressing with the clients, make sure you had access to the requisite paperwork or electronic resources; she would not ignore you or 'peer over your shoulder'. Meanwhile she would be managing her own workload effectively, something which Deirdre in the scenario appears unable to do.

The use of Deirdre as a mentor in the scenario is also an interesting management decision, because it is clear from the comments of others that Deirdre may not be popular with her colleagues. So what is the rationale for this decision? Some possibilities are as follows.

- Deirdre is the most senior midwife on duty and thus it is reasonable to assume she can cope with a new staff member.
- Deirdre's work is being made especially difficult, as a form of bullying.
- Deirdre is failing to work to her expected capacity or grade and she is being assessed by the manager.
- The manager is testing you out, by setting you to work with a difficult member of the staff.

It may well be that the manager herself has some competing priorities and is revealing them in this way; unfortunately this is putting you as the mentee in a difficult position. In particular, if a worker is failing to perform as expected, a manager may wish to observe that person in a particular situation, as part of an assessment.

Patient priorities

In Chapter 7 we saw that the deterioration of a patient requires recognition and then action, through effective communication. We will now consider patient dependence and how it affects working practices. For many years the staffing levels of clinical areas have reflected, to some extent, patient dependence levels and this possibly reflects medical intervention, rather than nursing care.

For instance, in an intensive care unit, where patients are critically ill, unconscious and requiring artificial ventilation, staffing levels are set at one-to-one for trained staff. In the delivery suite the midwife is also working one-to-one with the mother in labour and this is as it should be. In both situations there are multiple observations and interventions required and considerable risk to the client.

Now consider the step-down unit from intensive care or the delivery suite: this has clients who are less critically ill but who are also potentially confused or anxious. It is very unlikely that this area will have one-to-one trained staff and yet there may be a considerable amount of care needed.

You may work in an area where staff have had a skill mix review or one where there has been a reduction in the number of senior-grade staff.

The government has defined levels of care, with descriptors of what this means in patient terms (Department of Health, 2000a, cited by Creed and Spiers, 2010):

- level 0: patients whose needs can be met through normal ward care in an acute hospital;
- level 1: patients at risk of their condition deteriorating or those recently relocated from higher levels of care whose needs can be met on an acute ward with advice and support;
- level 2: patients requiring more detailed observation or intervention, including support for single-organ failure, postoperative care and those stepping down from higher levels of care;
- level 3: patients requiring advanced respiratory support or basic respiratory support and support of at least two other organs, including all complex patients requiring support for multiorgan failure.

Government is always trying to save costs and, as staffing budgets make up a vast amount of NHS costs, this is an area under review. There is no doubt that this sounds like a political issue, and it is; the move is to replace highly skilled and expensive staff with an equal number of less skilled and thus less expensive staff. It is clear that level 3 patients need to be in an intensive care setting, but level 1 and 2 patients might be on a general medical or surgical ward, without specialist-skilled staff. Assessing patient dependence and matching this to the staffing skill mix has long been a challenge and the development of a formula to assess this accurately has been a goal, but no two days in most healthcare settings are identical. Using the patient dependence levels to assess staffing levels and hence actual workload changes so much each day that it is hard to estimate the requirements of staffing a day, let alone three to four weeks, in advance, when the off-duty rota is written.

Setting priorities in a crisis

As a team leader, you have to work with the staff on duty at that time, regardless of patient dependence, so this what can you do.

1 Don't panic, as it does not help. Briefly talk to whatever staff you have about priorities.
2 If there is clearly a high risk to the patients in your care you must inform your line manager, ideally in writing, but a verbal message followed later by a written one is one way forward. By alerting your manager that the anticipated staffing levels on the shift have not been met, due to illness or other reasons, you are identifying a potential risk. The manager will attempt to find you staff, but you should also make use of junior staff or administrative staff to try and

obtain others, possibly from the pool of your own staff or the nursing bank. As you are the experienced staff member you are needed with the patients, not on the telephone, so delegate effectively and get feedback on the outcomes.

3   Identify those patients at immediate risk, for instance those with diabetes mellitus who need food or patients with important medication that can't be delayed. Either delegate these tasks, or if this isn't possible, do them yourself quickly.

4   Close the ward to admissions; this will affect medical staff and other departments and is likely to get the situation noticed quickly. Or if you have patients in the theatre suite, refuse to allow them to return: staffing levels in the recovery area are likely to be better.

5   Finally, and perhaps key, talk to your patients, tell them what you can't do and meet their important needs. For instance, making beds and giving washes aren't really important, even if they usually take up much of the shift; today they can wait, but taking a patient to the toilet and altering the position of someone with restricted movement are important.

At the end of the shift or if extra staff arrive, make a point of thanking those who have worked extra hard or differently from usual. Appreciation is a really important commodity, and a free one, not always used enough.

Later, when all is calm, review how the situation arose, and whether it could have been predicted or prevented. Clearly a sudden outbreak of an infectious disease, such as norovirus, might cause this to occur, but in this case the patients are probably affected as well and the ward must be closed. However, if this is not the case, could the staffing levels and skill mix have been predicted as potentially unsafe?

Management through the duty rota

Activity 8.6   *Decision-making*

How is the off-duty rota prepared where you work? Are there carefully controlled parameters or does it seem far from organised?

There is guidance on this activity at the end of the chapter.

A manager should have the priority of the 'on-duty' rather than the off-duty: the first reflects a concern for the resources needed for the task, the second approach concern for people. In reality, as staff are the resource, they have to be accommodated in a manner that suits them, but not in a way that can lead to a potentially unsafe situation. For instance, consider these questions, which are fundamental to a satisfactory staffing rota; if the answers are no, then this must be addressed.

*   Does the shift pattern ensure that there is sufficient time to hold an effective handover of care, or are staff always required to stay beyond their shift and do overtime?

*   Is there a requirement for a minimum number of registered or untrained staff on duty or does it vary from day to day?

*   How many staff can be on leave or on study days at the same time? Again, is grading factored into this?

- What grade of staff provides team leadership or does this vary?
- If there are a Sister/charge nurse and Junior Sister on the staffing, do they perform different roles or just work opposite shifts?
- Are the supernumerary students always allocated to work the same shifts as their mentors?

Activity 8.7   *Leadership and managememt*

You are required to complete the staff rota for the fortnight beginning 15 March.

Shift patterns are identified as follows:

> Long day (LD): 7.00a.m.–8.30p.m. (12.5 hours)
> Late (L): 1.30p.m.–9.30p.m. (7.5 hours)
> Early (E): 7.00a.m.–3p.m. (7.5 hours)
> Night (N): 8.00p.m.–7.30a.m. (10.5 hours)
> Late half (LH): 2p.m.–8.30p.m. (6 hours)
> Early half (EH) 7a.m.–1.30p.m. (6 hours)
> Part-time (PT): works 15 hours a week

Other abbreviations included on the rota include: S/D, study day; DO_R, day off, requested by staff member; EH_R, early half, requested by staff member; and S, sick.

Rota criteria

- Full-time shift is 37.5 hours a week (75 hours a fortnight).
- Matron and nurse practitioner (NP) Nick Cameron work late/early shifts Monday to Friday and do not do night shifts.
- Healthcare assistant (HCA) Wright only works weekends.
- HCA Riley does not work long days.
- For clinical safety, two qualified members of staff have to be on duty on each shift.
- On nights there need to be at least three members of staff on duty.
- All students are supernumerary but have to complete the equivalent of 37.5 hours of practice per week unless on university days.
- Matron is the mentor for student nurse (St/n) Fletcher; staff nurse (SN) Buckingham is the mentor for St/n Black; SN Robinson is the mentor for St/n Wyatt; SN Mustafa is the mentor for St/n Cohen.

Rota information

- SN Buckingham has S/D Monday 15 and Tuesday 16.
- HCA Laverty is off on planned sick for the w/c 15/3 (back 22/3).
- HCA Ben Wright has a study day on Friday 26.
- SN Steve Robinson has requested the weekend of 20–21 off to attend a wedding.
- SN Sarah Grimshaw has requested that she should not do night duty during the first half of the rota.

continued . . .

- HCA Maxine Blair has requested the weekend off on 27–28 (no reason given).
- HCA Paul Brown has requested an EH on Monday 22 for a dental appointment.
- Matron has requested she works three shifts with St/n Fletcher as she is due to sign off her placement this week (St/n Fletcher leaves 21/3).
- St/n Nicholas Wyatt is on a study week w/c 22/3.
- St/n Jim Cohen has study days Thursday 18 and Friday 19.

Name and grade	Mon	Tues	Wednes	Thurs	Fri	Sat	Sun
Totals							
a.m.							
p.m.							
Night							

There is a sample solution at the end of the chapter.

Patient priorities in the community

Scenario

The scene has shifted to the community midwifery team, where there has been more than the usual number of new mothers in the area. In particular, many are not English-speaking, having come from Eastern Europe in the last two years. In the hospital setting there is a midwife fluent in Polish and a midwifery care assistant who speaks some Romanian, but there is no one in the community with these language skills. Although you are now working on rotation between the hospital and the community, you are still only doing two long day shifts a week. This, coupled with the language barrier, means you know there are going to be problems communicating with these families, and you are not sure what will happen on your occasional visits.

The inability to communicate directly with a client is one of the most taxing care situations; relying on interpreters is far from ideal and can lead to accidental and sometimes purposeful misunderstanding or misinterpretation. You are fortunate because the trust can assist you in this situation, as each mother has been given a 'frequently asked questions' sheet with the Polish or Romanian translations written beneath each statement. When you first visit one of these mothers it seems unnatural to have to rely on a sheet of paper to guide your discussions. You are soon able to combine your observations with the question sheet to provide some satisfactory and safe outcomes; however you would much rather have a native speaker with you.

As you continue through the shift it is mid-afternoon, when you are phoned and asked to make an urgent visit to a mother-to-be on the other side of town, but you have just arrived outside the house of one of your planned visits. The planned visit has already been put back from early this morning, when you had arranged to meet. This is a real question of priorities. Can you delegate or ask someone else to visit the other woman? Should you cancel this planned visit yet again, as you may not be able to return here, if the urgency is real?

You decide to make a few important phone calls, one back to your base and another to the urgent visit, rather than just rushing onwards with either. The phone call to base reveals that the urgent visit is for a woman, possibly in labour with her first child, who is known to be very anxious and whom you have met once before and who is Romanian. You ask if anyone is free to visit instead of you and are told that the only person available and close to the client is the care assistant. You ring the care assistant and ask her to go to the client; you ring the client and inform her of your short delay and also about the Romanian-speaking midwifery care assistant calling in immediately. You really hope that whoever answers your phone call will have a good level of English; fortunately it is the neighbour who quickly understands what will happen. You know that the care assistant will recognise a real emergency and quickly phone 999 for an ambulance if needed and with the advantage of a shared language may identify any particular issues.

continued . . .

> You make your planned visit, apologising for the delay, and are able to offer some breast-feeding advice to the new mother, who was feeling concerned about her baby's milk intake. You would like to stay and chat more to offer real support, which you feel is needed here, but decline the offered cup of coffee, stating that you have just had one. You make another appointment to come back tomorrow for a longer visit, with the excuse of checking on the breast-feeding, and rush to the other client.

Prioritising and delegating

This is a situation both of competing priorities and appropriate delegation, which you have managed effectively. First, by taking a short time to understand the issue, you were able to ascertain the urgency of the problem with the Romanian mother-to-be and provide a temporary solution, to identify quickly if an emergency existed. Leaving your original client without her overdue visit could have meant missing a serious problem with the mother or the baby. The quick visit has assured both the mother and yourself that the issues of feeding were not too serious and if the mother takes your advice the visit tomorrow may be to a more relaxed family.

Personal time management

Planning ahead is very important with today's busy lifestyle, whether it is at home or work. Very few of us have time to waste; even our leisure time can be busy. Let's go back to the scenario at the start of the chapter, where your partner hadn't prepared a meal as you had asked, to await your return home on your first day. In this situation you might be angry unless an alternative solution was presented, such as a meal out or take-away as a celebration. On the days when you are working a long day, expecting to prepare a meal afterwards may be unrealistic, but so is getting take-away every night you work, both on health and financial grounds.

Many mature students or those embarking on further studies, or changes in their working week, expect to be able to cope regardless of however many challenges are made of them. If you had a busy life between work and home, prior to undertaking a study module, where will you find the extra time? The key is to decide on the priorities and possibly give something up, at least temporarily, to free up some time.

The sort of time-saving tips that you find in magazines do make sense and can really help you manage some of your time. Examples include the following.

- When you cook a meal, make several portions and freeze some.
- Set up a slow cooker with cheap ingredients to cook to tender during the working day.
- Use a shopping list to save time and avoid overspending; shop on the way home to save a separate journey.
- Make packed lunches the night before; this saves both money and time.

Working effectively and efficiently means you save time, time which can be spent either as you wish at home or improving other aspects of care at work. Completing a task properly the first time is an approach to quality management that attempts to remove mistakes and errors.

Clinical governance

In the health service quality assurance is frequently called clinical governance (see Chapter 7), perhaps reflecting the difficult nature of the 'product' in healthcare. Clinical quality is much harder to define than the quality of an electrical gadget as there are very many perspectives on the quality of health; after all the NHS really manages ill health, not health, as far less money is expended on prevention than on treatment.

In the manufacturing industry, good quality means making it right first time every time and thus avoiding waste. For instance, you may buy a particular relatively expensive brand of baked beans, because you believe it will always be eaten and never wasted, whereas a cheap brand is rejected and wasted and thus is more expensive in the long run.

Other views of quality are that the higher the price, the better the quality; although many consumers believe that high cost and exclusivity automatically equate to high quality, it might not. For example, if there are two 'identical' products, where one is brand-name and the other a supermarket own brand, the brand-named product may not be superior: it may just be that the branded product has higher manufacturing costs, not better ingredients or components.

There is another view that some items are high-quality because we are told they are and we come to believe it. This is very clearly illustrated by the use of logos and branded products that some teenagers will only accept, to the exclusion of any other comparable product.

Finally there is the consumer view that a product must be fit for purpose and meet expectations, which seems more realistic; but assessing those expectations is much more difficult.

If healthcare quality were as simple as any other product, then paying for a branded (or non-NHS) service or treatment might deliver higher quality. The problem with health, as a product, is that what we actually want are services that prevent ill health, such as screening services; services that meet our increasing expectations, such as providing infertility treatment; and services that provide cutting-edge life-saving treatment – and all at minimal cost.

Activity 8.8   *Critical thinking*

How do you judge the health services available for you and your family? Do these judgments differ when you are a worker rather than a user?

There is guidance on this activity at the end of the chapter.

McSherry and Pearce (2002, p12) defined clinical governance as *guaranteeing clinical quality improvement at all levels of healthcare provision* and it can be traced back to *The New NHS: Modern, Dependable* (Department of Health, 1997). Clinical governance was developed from corporate governance, identifying the way companies ought to behave, with clear financial dealings, efficient and effective operations and compliance with the law. In each corporation a chief executive takes responsibility for the actions of the organisation, in its dealings with shareholders and the public. McSherry and Pearce go on to state that clinical governance in the health service requires an organisation to have an environment which supports and values its staff, promotes individual accountability, aims to improve and maintain quality processes and promotes safe practice (standard setting and risk management).

In the context of your work this has been translated into things such as:

- staff appraisal, staff development and mandatory training;
- record keeping and Criminal Records Bureau checks and professional registration;
- implementation of policies and procedures, from government and national advisory services, at local level;
- risk assessments that have been carried out to ensure safe working practices for staff, visitors and patients, e.g. moving and handling training, fire and safety training or Control of Substances Hazardous to Health.

Activity 8.9   *Communication*

Study one local policy that has been implemented in your clinical area and find out the underpinning clinical recommendations or government directive.

No outline answer is given for this activity.

The current accepted definition of clinical audit appears in *Principles for Best Practice in Clinical Audit* (NICE, CHI and RCN, 2002) and was endorsed by the National Institute of health and Clinical Excellence (NICE):

> *Clinical audit is a quality improvement process that seeks to improve patient care and outcomes through systematic review of care against explicit criteria and the implementation of change. Aspects of the structure, process and outcome of care are selected and systematically evaluated against explicit criteria. Where indicated changes are implemented at an individual, team, or service level and further monitoring is used to confirm improvement in healthcare delivery.*

Alternatively, and more simply, *audit involves improving the quality of patient care by looking at current practice and modifying it where necessary* (**www.clinicalauditsupport.com/what_is_clinical_audit.html**).

Clinical governance should therefore not be about completing paperwork to prove that an activity has been undertaken, nor should it be about a department following up complaints, although both are important in their way. It should be about getting it right first time every time. An episode of treatment and its outcome should be as expectedly successful as the purchase of a tin of your favourite baked beans! Patients shouldn't acquire pressure sores while in a care setting and they shouldn't become malnourished – both of which, tragically, still happen (Healthcare Quality Improvement Partnership, 2011).

The demands of the budget

One area not yet touched on is the competing demands of financial pressures. You are used to managing your own financial burdens, but what about those at work? It is likely that your only encounter with financial issues is the constraint of not filling vacant posts or providing different clinical products to save money.

Scenario

Your unit manager has organised a meeting with all the staff to explain that cuts need to be made within your ward, to the equivalent of one trained midwife. She explains that she can transfer money between budgets as long as the overall expenditure is reduced (Woodhall and Stuttard, 1999). She wants you all, as a team, to look at the way this money might be saved instead of simply failing to fill the up-coming vacancy. The manager explains that there will be no incremental increase in any of the wards' budgets this year, yet costs will continue to rise, so savings must be made. The meeting is at risk of deteriorating into a criticism of the trust until one of your colleagues points out that you are all being asked to consider a better way of working.

A budget is an amount of money allocated to a manager for a specific purpose and time period, so budget management should have clarity, timing, focus, action and reaction if it is to work effectively. A manager will have many different budgets but they all finally result in the unit cost. So, taking a factory situation, what must also be remembered is that as more items are produced, for instance toasters (patients treated), the total cost of producing all the toasters (patients treated) will rise. This is because each toaster (patient) uses new components that have to be purchased, so overall there is more expenditure on components. However the fixed costs, those associated with running the factory or hospital, such as the heating bill or the cost of permanent staff, remain the same. So as the number of toasters made (or patients treated) increases, the proportion of fixed costs applied to each toaster (patient) falls and hence the average costs of each toaster (patient) fall and thus profit should rise (Bryans, 2005). In a non-profit-making health environment, profit is replaced by doing more for the same money.

Financial issues are not ones that most junior nurses think about, yet costs and expenditure impinge on everyone all the time. The central issue in healthcare finances is driving down costs, through better ways of working and getting more services for less or equivalent costs. In addressing the questions in the final scenario you need to know the actual costs to be saved and consider all ways to save money, because the savings are likely to come in a variety of smaller ways. The following issues might be considered.

- Does the off-duty have peaks and troughs in staffing levels, and if so, could these be levelled out by changing shift patterns, while maintaining quality?
- Are bank or agency staff employed frequently, also reflecting poor off-duty planning?
- Are clinical stores being wasted because no one knows the actual cost of the items?

- Is medication managed effectively?
- Are paper and printing costs for the unit unrealistic?

Overall, in the same way that you manage your home finances, the clinical unit manager must manage those of the ward or area. The more involvement and understanding you have of financial issues, the more you will be able to understand the need for good-quality management. Getting care right the first time saves money as well as patient distress.

Activities: brief outline answers

Activity 8.3

Your reflections should have revolved around the ability of individuals to function maximally at all times and how tiredness might impair this. Nurses seem to have a real problem with taking breaks, particularly as they feel an earlier finish time is better. Unfortunately, missing a break regularly can be detrimental, even if finishing earlier is more convenient in terms of travel or child care. Planning breaks into the day, from the start, can be really helpful and indicates concern for both the team and the workload.

Activity 8.4

Here are some of your potential uses of time.

The time just went by without any conscious activity.

I spent time 'firefighting' a crisis which could have been averted.

I had to chat to someone; I am always a good listener and happy to hear problems, but I got diverted from the task in hand.

I had to chair a meeting, but it didn't start or finish on time and the minutes will be late being sent out.

I forgot my shopping or 'to do' list; and so didn't buy everything or achieve the priority.

Activity 8.5

If it is away, why do you do this and do you ever have to go back to the client to clarify a detail?

If you sit in the office with colleagues doing paperwork, do you get side-tracked and talk about other issues?

If you are by the bedside, do you have access to all the available data?

Do you write the same information more than once in documents?

All these activities waste time.

Activity 8.6

If you have never really thought about how the off-duty is constructed, this is your opportunity to have a look at the rota where you work. Try to notice peaks and troughs in staffing numbers or grades; does this reflect no workload differences? Are the grades of staff being used appropriately? Are students always rostered with their mentor or buddy mentor? Are there patterns of sickness and absenteeism?

Activity 8.7

Name and grade	Mon 15th	Tues 16th	Wed 17th	Thur 18th	Fri 19th	Sat 20th	Sun 21st	Mon 22nd	Tues 23rd	Wed 24th	Thurs 25th	Fri 26th	Sat 27th	Sun 28th	hours
Matron	E	L	L	E	E	DO	DO	L	E	E	L	L	DO	DO	75
NP Cameron	L	E	E	L	L	DO	DO	E	L	L	E	E	DO	DO	75
SN Buckingham	S/D	S/D	DO	DO	DO	LD	LD	N	N	DO	DO	DO	E	EH	74.50
SN Grimshaw	DO	DO	EH	EH	DO	LD	LD	DO	EH	N	N	N	DO	DO	74.50
SN Mustafa	DO	DO	DO	N	N	N	N	DO	DO	LD	LD	LD	DO	DO	79.50
SN Robinson	N	N	N	DO	EH	DO$_R$	DO$_R$	LD	DO	DO	DO	DO	L	L	77.5
Bank SN(s)	LD	LD	LH	LH	LH								N	L&N	72
St/n Fletcher	E	>	>	>	>	DO	DO	left	>	>	>	>	>	>	
St/n Black	L	E	DO	DO	L	E	E	N	N	DO	DO	DO	E	E	37.5
St/n Cohen	DO	DO	DO	S/D	S/D	N	N	DO	DO	LD	LD	LD	DO	DO	73.5
St/n Wyatt	N	N	N	DO	LH	DO	DO	study	week	>	>	>	>	>	37.5
Bank HCA(s)				LH & N	N	N	>	N	N	N	N	N	N	N	79.5
HCA Laverty	sick	>	>	>	>	>	>	DO	DO	DO	N	N	N	N	42
HCA Blair	LD	LD	LD	DO	DO	DO	DO	N	N	N	DO	EH	DO$_R$	DO$_R$	75
HCA Brown	DO	DO$_R$	DO	N	N	N	N	EH$_R$	LD	E	L	DO	DO$_R$	DO$_R$	75.5
HCA Riley	N	N	N	DO	EH	DO	DO	L	E	L	E	E	DO	DO	75
HCA Wright						L	L	L	E	L	E	S/D	DO	L	30
Totals															
a.m.	3 + 1	3+1	3	3	3	3	3	3	4	4	4	4	2+1	2+1	
p.m.	3+1	3+1	3+1	1+2	3+1	3	3	3	3	4	4	3	1+2	2+1	
Nights	3	3	3	2+1	2+1	3	3	3	3	2+1	2+1	2+1	1+2	1+2	

Activity 8.8

Your expectations from the health service will be affected by issues as diverse as your social situation, age, sex, cultural background and wealth. So you may have expectations about infertility treatment, free dental care or quick access to orthopaedic surgery.

Further reading and useful websites

Stress tests can be found at Life Stressor Tests on: **www.cliving.org/lifestresstestscore.htm**

or at Rudebusters on **www.rudebusters.com/stresqwz.htm**

If you want to read more about absenteeism and the workforce try:

benefits.org/interface/cost/absent2.htm

http://www.softworks-workforce.com/ie/

If you want to read more about financial management and budgeting, try:

www.ncvo-vol.org.uk/advice-support/funding-finance/financial-management

Chapter 9
What if someone wants to make a complaint?

Chapter aims

After reading this chapter, you will be able to:

- analyse the probable causes when things go wrong;
- appreciate the importance of assessing a broad picture in patient care, rather than just the details;
- follow through a patient or family complaint;
- understand the importance of avoiding errors that lead to complaints.

Introduction

This chapter is about quality assurance, and focuses on a scenario about a complaint of poor care and poor nutrition in a community hospital. We will look at the issues of care, compassion and escalating concerns (NMC, 2010; Commission for Quality Care: **www.cqc.org.uk/**) to more senior staff.

In Chapter 8 we looked at the theory behind quality, arising as it did from industrial models, as well as how you might manage competing priorities in practice. This chapter will build on this by considering what can, nevertheless, go wrong, and what to do when things do go wrong. Most importantly, the outcome should be that you consider carefully the practice where you work and how to avoid errors in the first place.

Grounds for complaint

Scenario

You are working in a community hospital, in a post that you enjoy, having been appointed after you registered last October. Today you are back on duty in mid-January after a fortnight's skiing holiday, a belated reward from your partner for qualifying. You happily worked over Christmas and new year, as your partner was also on call, and looked forward to your holiday. Over the Christmas period you admitted Joyce, a 78-year-old widow who had various medical problems, including a large venous ulcer. Her GP had liaised with the unit about her admission as her family had talked to him and the district nursing team about the worsening ulcer. Joyce has limited mobility due to arthritis as well as the leg ulcer, but her family had provided her with shopping and cooked meals. Both Joyce and her family hoped that, after a period as an inpatient, when her leg ulcer would improve, she would return to independence at home. Joyce enjoyed her meals and her body mass index (BMI) on admission indicated she was slightly overweight; and she freely admitted to having a weakness for chocolate biscuits, particularly if a proper meal wasn't available.

When you admitted Joyce, you talked about her family Christmas and she asked why you were working over the holidays. Joyce was a chatty person, keen to be as independent as possible, but able to understand and be compliant with her treatment. The specialist tissue viability team were making progress in treating the leg ulcer, which, coupled with bed rest, was making a marked difference to healing; you had expected that she would have been discharged home while you were away.

Meeting Joyce again after your holiday you are surprised to see her looking as if she has lost considerable weight; she looks rather unkempt and sad, so you go to talk with her at the first opportunity.

| Activity 9.1 | *Evidence-based practice and research* |

Why would Joyce's leg ulcer improve on the ward? Remind yourself of the factors influencing leg ulcer management.

There is guidance on this activity at the end of the chapter.

When admitting patients to a care area we frequently undertake a range of routine assessments including vital signs, urinalysis, height-to-weight ratio and BMI (NHS Choices, 2010), as well as more complex tests such as blood analysis, ECG or chest X-ray, to develop a baseline measure of health. All too frequently the findings from at least some of these tests are recorded without thought to their significance. This is certainly true of the acutely ill adult where a patient's deterioration has not been recognised quickly, hence the development and use of 'track and trigger' systems such as Early Warning System (EWS), Modified Early Warning System (MEWS) or ALERT (see Chapter 7). In Joyce's case, she was not acutely ill on admission and the routine screening tests really only revealed an elevated BMI, so there was no reason to expect deterioration in her health.

Scenario

The handover report mentioned that Joyce's leg ulcer was not really showing signs of improvement and that the social worker was investigating a nursing-home bed as she was not fit to return home. Joyce is clearly pleased to see you and promptly bursts into tears, so you sit down for a chat; the other staff can provide cover for your work for a few minutes. Joyce explains that one of the doctors, she isn't sure who, said she had to lose weight and so the dietician had visited. Low-calorie food had been organised with lots of salad, sugar had been banned from drinks and Joyce's intake was to be charted. Joyce admitted that she disliked the bitter aftertaste of sweetener and salad gave her indigestion, but she didn't like to complain and ask for anything else, as the dietician had been so insistent on her weight loss.

You note that a food chart has been instigated and it appears that Joyce is following her diet well, but when you ask her to confirm what she ate yesterday, she says not much. So you agree to come back after breakfast and discuss what is charted and what she has actually eaten. Unfortunately you can't check on Joyce's actual breakfast intake, but when you come back mid-morning her food chart indicates that she had apparently eaten. Joyce says she had a couple of spoonfuls of unsweetened porridge and the chart says porridge eaten, so there is clearly a discrepancy between interpretations of food consumed. You raise the issue at the team meeting later in the morning. The healthcare assistants (HCAs) comment that if Joyce is to lose weight then the less she eats the better, so they can see no problem with what is being recorded. They perceive that she is just not hungry and so not eating as much; it is clear that they have little understanding of the importance of a balanced diet in terms of health needs.

The use of charts and recording systems is only as effective as those using them. In this instance the food chart shouldn't just be a prompt for recording calorie intake or the lack of it, but also the quality of nutrition. A seminal work was written on the importance of good nutritional intake in hospital (Coates, 1985), then the *Essence of Care* (Department of Health, 2010b) documented similar issues and ways to improve the situation – 25 years later the Department of Health (2010b) is again discussing the poor diet of inpatients.

The NMC stresses the importance of documentation as an adjunct to accountability, which is correct; but this means that the documentation must also be accurate. Documentation should not be the measure of good nursing care; rather it should be a secondary consideration to follow actual care. Yet all too often paperwork seems to have taken over as the priority; clinical governance strategies aim to improve quality in healthcare, yet now gathering statistics is seen as paramount. Penalties are incurred when care targets are breached, and the reasons for this were excellent: patients shouldn't wait for 18 hours in A&E on a trolley because no one can find a bed. Yet surely they shouldn't be pushed on to an overcrowded ward, and left unattended there, just because a four-hour wait in A&E is going to be exceeded.

When you consider the way that quality assurance developed in the manufacturing industry, it wasn't through documentation: it was through careful attention to detail. It was management listening to what clients and shop floor workers said about the product and making sure that the product was fit for purpose. In the scenario, Joyce does need to get her weight down and being immobile in a hospital bed won't help burn calories, but the quality of her diet is important if her general health and the leg ulcer, in particular, are going to improve (not to mention her feeling of well-being).

Scenario

With a little thought and communication with the HCAs, dieticians and the catering team, Joyce's diet improves. She now receives small portions of a more varied diet, which she enjoys, and fruit replaces most of the much-missed chocolate biscuits. A couple of days later, you are informed that Joyce has been complaining of increased pain at the site of her leg ulcer, which also appears inflamed; a swab for microbial culture reveals methicillin-resistant *Staphylococcus aureus* (MRSA). The presence of this organism means that Joyce must be moved to a side ward as well as start antibiotic therapy.

The next day, Joyce's daughter, who has been increasingly concerned about her mother's health, brings in a letter of complaint, which is a copy of one sent to the consultant in charge of Joyce's care. She says that she feels you should know what is happening, as you have always helped her mother to get better, and she doesn't blame you.

Tragically, two weeks after being started on treatment for MRSA, and having developed *Clostridium difficile*, Joyce dies.

Activity 9.2	*Critical thinking*

What would you do, in response to this complaint?

An outline answer is provided at the end of the chapter.

Customer expectations

In industry, customer service is an important part of a company's operations, and when products or services are faulty, there is a system in place to deal with it. Manufacturing and other service industries have usually accepted that the 'customer is always right'. Medicine has taken a long time to catch up with this progress. The Patient's Charter (Department of Health, 1993) started to empower individuals and make them aware of what could reasonably be expected from healthcare providers and was delivered to all householders in the UK. It was the first move to treat patients like consumers of other products. The objectives of making patients aware of what was reasonable, and that choice did exist, were helpful, but concepts such as the 'named nurse' or waiting-time limits have put unreasonable pressures on healthcare providers.

Patients and clients now have internet access to good-quality healthcare research, such as the Cochrane Library, and are thus rightly knowledgeable about what they can expect from treatment. Unfortunately the demands on the system continue to rise, due both to an ageing and increasingly frail elderly population, and people's expectations. In parallel with this has been the growth of litigation, where individuals pursue healthcare providers for compensation, when expected outcomes aren't achieved. The most recent figures stated that in the year 2010–11 £3 million was paid out in compensation (UK Parliament, 2012) and claims continue to rise year on year.

When complaints about poor practice are being considered, the law will ask what 'reasonable behaviour' is, and will apply previous case law to judge the outcomes. In some high-profile cases, such as the Bristol Royal Infirmary inquiry into infant deaths or the high mortality rates for patients of the GP Dr Harold Shipman, the organisations as a whole were blamed as they didn't challenge medical practitioners and raise concerns. In other cases patients who can prove that they have suffered from a healthcare-acquired infection have successfully sued a trust for compensation.

Identifying failings

Returning to the scenario, how should you take this event forward? You will of course remain polite and courteous and thank the daughter for copying you into the letter. Would you ask if this can be shared with colleagues or your ward manager? It is useful to have this consent as it means you can discuss the situation in a bottom-up fashion, as it will also be handled top-down from the consultant. Do you think the subsequent death of Joyce will worsen the situation?

The evidence states that many complaints can be dealt with through an apology, an acknowledgement that things have gone wrong, and information on how the situation might be prevented in future. So first you need to consider where the situation went wrong with Joyce and second, how it might have been prevented. You might identify the following areas.

1. A BMI assessment indicates a height-to-weight ratio, not the full nutritional state of the client, so should not indicate a simple weight loss programme without more detailed consideration by a dietician (NHS Choices, 2010).
2. Joyce had large venous ulcers that were not responding to community care and may have been losing considerable amounts of serous fluid which has a high protein content. This would have resulted in Joyce needing additional protein intake.
3. Joyce's preferred meal pattern might be termed grazing, and so the three-meal pattern of hospital food will not have suited her; smaller, more frequent snacks would have been preferred.
4. Joyce is one of a number of people who can taste artificial sweetener as bitter.
5. As an elderly person, Joyce is from a generation that often accepts medical and nursing directives without question.
6. The communication to ensure the continuity of seamless care was flawed between the ward nurses, community staff, tissue viability team, GP and medical consultant, dietetic team, Joyce and her family.

Seeing the bigger picture

As a registered nurse you should be able to identify all these potential problems, because most will have been covered in your pre-registration programme. The problem is that they can't be seen in isolation, and that as a registered practitioner you must start to see the wider picture. Even though Joyce's diet isn't acceptable to her, she will not be able to challenge the 'prescription' because she will have been brought up to accept the medical decision without question. Joyce will be one of those patients who 'don't like to make a fuss' or feel the nurses are always too busy to bother. In this way Joyce's situation becomes progressively worse. No wonder she was pleased to see you.

At the root of most of Joyce's problems is poor communication between the multidisciplinary team (MDT), Joyce herself and her family. If her dietary requirements as a woman with severe leg ulcers (rather than with just a raised BMI), and her preferred eating patterns had been considered more fully, she might not have developed malnutrition. The lack of attention to hand hygiene by someone in the MDT probably resulted in cross-infection with MRSA. Staff still don't wash their hands between every patient contact, despite all the evidence that they should. Once colonised with MRSA, Joyce requires antibiotics and without good case management, including reference to prescribing protocols and infection control, *C. difficile* infection develops. The whole situation could have been avoidable if someone had looked at the bigger picture.

These realistic scenarios are intended to help you, the reader, visualise a situation as a fly on the wall, because once in practice we are all too often unable to stand back and consider what we are actually doing. When management gurus are sent into failing organisations, they look at the situation with an objective eye. Gerry Robinson, Mary Portas and Alex Polizzi (from various TV programmes) have been televised doing just this in the NHS, shops and hotels respectively, and then challenging the chief executive, owner or manager with what they find. Poor use of resources, poor use of people and poor communications are frequently at the root of the problem, although they are disguised in various ways.

If it's worth doing, do it properly

Nurses are frequently being encouraged to document everything (NMC, 2008b) to prove that the activities have been undertaken. However, the value of documentation is in the sharing of the information held there, so records should be accurate and honest. For instance, if the person completing a food intake chart doesn't know what Joyce actually eats at each of her meals, the chart is worse than useless – it is actually harmful.

How many times have you seen urine output on fluid balance charts recorded as 'out to toilet or incontinent ++'? Or the oral intake side of the chart completed by asking the patient, at the end of the day, how many cups of tea she had? Why bother with these charts? Look at the bigger picture. Is it important to know accurately about someone's fluid balance? If it is, then get it right. Try never to 'go through the motions' with record-keeping. Reflect the quality adage: 'get it right first time, every time'.

There is every reason to suppose that most of the time when fluid charts are filled in by guesswork, or patients don't get the right meals, these occurrences are not seen as errors. Errors are seen as something much more serious. Cass (2006), in her insightful book *The NHS Experience: The snakes and ladders' guide for patients and professionals,* writes about what causes people to make errors when they care for patients. She points out that it is because we are human and thus fallible that we make errors and that they will never be prevented. She comments that all we can do is try to work out when errors happen and reduce the chances of them happening.

Scenario

You are a staff nurse working on a busy medical admissions ward on a Saturday night, and you are buddy mentoring Jon, a third-year student nurse, on his penultimate placement. You have attended a course about intravenous (IV) drug administration and were deemed competent some months ago. IV drug administration is a skill you use frequently and with confidence.

Mrs Jones has been on the ward for three hours now; she is an oncology patient, whose permanent IV port has become inflamed. The F2 doctor (see Chapter 1) has seen Mrs Jones and prescribed antibiotics, and inserted another form of venous access in the patient's foot; the antibiotic is a new drug only recently prescribed in the hospital. At the prescribed time you and Jon go to the treatment room to prepare the antibiotic. The hospital policy requires that the nurse who administers the drug draws up the dose, and does not need a second person to check the prescription. Jon asks if he can draw up the drug, under supervision. The dose is written as 100mg in 10ml of water; you allow Jon to draw up the drug and he pays attention to asepsis at all times.

continued . . .

You go to Mrs Jones and check the patient against the prescription and administer the IV drug slowly over one minute. Mrs Jones says that it feels cold and stings a bit but you administer the whole dose and sign the prescription chart, after flushing with normal saline.

The following day the IV site in the foot is inflamed and the skin around the site has become discoloured, with Mrs Jones complaining of pain. It is apparent that the drug has entered the tissues around the site, causing severe damage.

You are called to see the ward manager and asked what happened when you gave the drug. The patient has refused to have any more antibiotic, either through the IV site in the foot or elsewhere.

Activity 9.3   *Critical thinking*

Where do you think things went wrong?

The answer to this activity is discussed below.

There are a number of places where this drug administration went wrong which may have accounted for the problem.

1. The F2 doctor didn't check with the on-call pharmacist about prescribing this drug and the correct dilution, as had been advised in a recent memo.
2. The F2 doctor should not have prescribed the drug to be administered via a peripheral IV line, as it was known to be an irritant.
3. The drug was not known to the staff nurse and, although 100mg seemed a reasonable dose for an antibiotic, this should have been checked.
4. The student diluted the drug with 10ml of water for injections. Without checking the *British National Formulary*, he wouldn't have known that it should have been diluted to 100ml and that water for injections also had to be used for the IV flush to prevent any interaction.
5. The patient's concerns weren't listened to at the time.
6. The hospital policy for administration of IV drugs was broken.

Cass suggest the following causes of errors (Cass, 2006, p138), all of which can be considered to have occurred in the scenario (Figure 9.1).

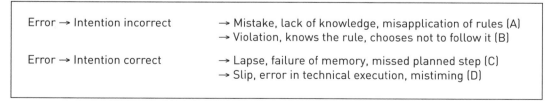

Error → Intention incorrect	→ Mistake, lack of knowledge, misapplication of rules (A)
	→ Violation, knows the rule, chooses not to follow it (B)
Error → Intention correct	→ Lapse, failure of memory, missed planned step (C)
	→ Slip, error in technical execution, mistiming (D)

Figure 9.1. Causes of errors.

The first mistake (point 1) is an example of D; the doctor was intent on prescribing correctly but made an error by not checking with pharmacy, as was advised in a memo. The doctor had prescribed an appropriate antibiotic for this patient, but would have been reminded by the pharmacist about dilution.

If the doctor had contacted the pharmacy (point 2), information about the correct dilution would have been passed to the staff nurse. She would have recognised that a 100ml injection could not have been administered by bolus injection, but would have required a small infusion, an example of (C).

The next issue (3) is where the staff nurse does not apply the rules (A) fundamental to safe drug administration, which is always to research any unfamiliar drug through the *British National Formulary*; she didn't apply the rule.

Finally, involving the student in drawing up the drug (4) violates the trust rule (B). As a buddy mentor the staff nurse is keen for the student to learn, but is distracted from following safe practice because her attention is being given to supervising the student. Finally, if patients exhibit unusual symptoms or remark that the medicine is different, this should act a spur to checking for safe practice.

This scenario is a set of mistakes, which singly would probably not have led to patient harm, because at each stage a check would have rectified the problem. Cass (2006, citing Reason, 2000) considers this series of effects to be like slices of Swiss Emmental cheese: each slice represents an element of practice or part of a procedure, with a number of holes through which poor practice can slip. So organisations put in place policies and procedures which attempt to limit the number of holes (risk points) and, in particular, prevent the holes from lining up between each slice. If the holes all line up, the error is not detected until it harms the patient.

Quality assurance is thus not just about getting the product right first time, every time, but also about not making errors. Clinical governance was established under the 1999 Health Act to create an environment that would strive to improve quality continually. It had seven pillars or domains of activity (Talbot-Smith and Pollock, 2006):

1. clinical audit, to measure performance against best practice;
2. clinical risk management with policies aimed at reducing risk;
3. clinical effectiveness programmes using National Service Frameworks or the guidance from the National Institute for Health and Clinical Excellence (NICE) to consider ways of working;
4. education and continued professional development of staff to ensure that staff are up to date;
5. staffing and staff management, including human relations policies and appraisal processes;
6. the use of IT to gather information and disseminate findings;
7. patient involvement in service planning – from this developed the Patient Advice and Liaison Services (PALS).

Clinical governance in the health service should thus look at procedures and, more importantly, at errors and try to find out why they occurred. The aerospace and nuclear power industries developed the idea of looking carefully at errors and near-misses to analyse why they happened (Cass, 2006, citing Barach and Small, 2000). For instance, if two airplanes come far too close to each other but there isn't a collision, staff will investigate why this potential accident arose. This culture of looking for causes rather than for someone to blame has taken a long time to establish itself in the health service, where traditionally an individual was blamed personally for any mistake. The Department of Health (2000b) produced the paper *An Organisation with a Memory* which aimed to direct staff to consider critical incidents and thus try to identify and remove risk factors.

Here are two examples of this in practice. In the past, if a patient required the administration of intravenous potassium, the nurse would be required to add a small concentrated amount to a larger volume. This was a hazardous procedure, as when incorrectly mixed a lethal bolus could occur. To avoid this, it is now normal procedure to provide potassium ready-diluted in other larger quantities of IV fluids.

Feed for administration via a nasogastric tube was confused with IV fluids as they appeared similar and the giving sets/syringes were interchangeable, resulting in patient death. One simple strategy, to avoid injecting oral fluids intravenously, is that syringes designed for oral use cannot be fitted to IV systems; others are coloured purple as a warning.

Large numbers of texts are available to consider in more depth the legal issues and accountability (Dimond, 2011) and these illustrate both the problems and the legal outcomes. In practice when things go wrong, patients quite reasonably want apologies. The evidence is that patients and their relatives do understand that errors can happen, but that a wall of silence or sometimes the suggestion that it was the patient's own fault only leads to anger. Patients and their families want an apology and they want to understand how it happened so it won't happen again. So, in any situation involving a complaint, Cass (2006) suggests the following type of process should be followed.

1. Document the occurrence carefully and clearly, noting only the facts and without supposition; note the time of events and, if equipment is involved, remove it from use or bag it up.
2. Meet the patient or family at a time that is convenient to them and apologise without blame.
3. Have a third party there who is impartial leading the meeting to avoid anger, PALS team members can help as advocates for the family. The organisation's legal team should have been informed.
4. Take comprehensive notes of the meeting and ensure the patient or family has a copy of them and agrees that they are an accurate record.
5. Note clearly what the family wants to happen and take all steps to do this to reassure the family that appropriate action has been taken regarding staff or equipment. Staff also have a right to confidentiality so individuals who are facing disciplinary procedures don't have to be named.

Escalating concerns

The Department of Health wants all complaints resolved locally if possible, but the CQC is now the overall reviewer of care providers. Individuals, patient's families, members of the public or professionals can contact the CQC anonymously and ask that a healthcare facility be reviewed. The CQC is responsible for a vast number of health and social care providers; it reported in

January 2012 on the four key areas relating to care providers (**www.cqc.org.uk/media/ people-often-not-centre-their-own-care-says-cqc-it-publishes-reports-its-review- services-people**). These were: (1) the shape of health and social care provision; (2) access to care services; (3) choices and control for patients; and (4) quality and safety. It noted that there were 140,000 inpatient beds in the NHS, 2,500 independent hospitals, 2,608 nursing homes, 13,475 care homes and 5,894 providers of domiciliary care. From these numbers it is clear that there are very many areas where patients and clients are at risk from harm, intentional or otherwise. So everyone, professional or otherwise, must ensure that incidents are always reported and acted on and where necessary the CQC is made aware of problem areas.

Activities: brief outline answers

Activity 9.1

Did you consider the importance of issues associated with general health, rather than specific wound care regimes? Did you remember about the diagnostic tests for arterial or venous ulcers and their subsequent treatment?

Activity 9.2

Would you get angry and deny any responsibility? After all, you were on leave for much of Joyce's stay on the ward; or you might blame it on the HCAs. Or would you apologise on behalf of the hospital and assure the family that you will pass the letter to your manager?

You should also have considered if the MRSA infection could have been prevented.

What about Joyce's subsequent death; could this have been prevented?

Further reading and useful websites

Go online and watch one of *The Fixer* programmes with Alex Polizzi, and her approach to turning around failing small business.

Watch **www.bbc.co.uk/programmes/b01bnd19** or any of the others in *The Fixer* series. You will notice areas like team work, feedback and customer need.

To enhance your knowledge of patient nutrition, read the following:

Coates, V (1985) *Are they Being Served? An investigation into the nutritional care given by nurses to acute medical patients and the influence of ward organisational patterns on that care.* London: Royal College of Nursing.

Salvage, J and Scott, C (2005) *Patients' nutritional care in hospital: an ethnographic study of nurses' role and patients' experience.* London: Royal College of Nursing.

www.rcn.org.uk/

The RCN website provides more resources on patient nutrition.

www.bapen.org.uk/musttoolkit.html

The malnutrition screening tool is available through BAPEN.

www.cqc.org.uk/standards

Essential standards for healthcare providers can be found through the CQC online.

Chapter 10
Developing your career: is there a perfect route?

Introduction

This chapter considers how you can influence your future career, through the effective use of past experience. The scenario involves the consideration of a job application and how you can demonstrate the skills for a new post.

Students often ask about how their carers should progress, in particular if their first job post-registration is not the one they wanted. Throughout this book, the scenarios have been set in areas where the nurse is pleased to be working, but in reality this doesn't always happen. So this chapter will consider career development at a time of financial crisis and of high unemployment. It will start by looking at traditional issues such as curriculum vitae (CV) and applications, but move on to other areas such as continued registration and career pathways.

Transferable skills

Scenario

After completing your pre-registration programme, you had no option but to accept a post at a local nursing home. You had always imagined yourself in A&E and your placement as a second-year student had done nothing but reinforce your determination. So it was with great regret, and a desperate bank balance, that you accepted the only available local job, in a nursing home. To be fair, the post which you have been in for six months has been better than you imagined it would be as the staff are fun to be around. You have also been able to spend considerably more time caring for some patients than you would have in the NHS. Now you have seen an advertisement in your local paper for a Band 5 nurse in A&E, with experience, and as this is your dream job you want to apply. You e-mail the trust, as the advertisement requests, for an online application form and start to think about what you will write.

That evening your best friend rings and invites you out for a drink; he too has seen the advertisement and is currently working in the intensive therapy unit (ITU) covering a maternity leave position. You ask if he has the application form yet and wonder whether there is any point trying to compete with his application, let alone the many others.

Activity 10.1	*Reflection*

If this had been you in the scenario, what would you feel you had gained in this nursing home post? Make some notes on the benefits to your career.

An outline answer is provided at the end of the chapter.

During your pre-registration programme, you will have encountered lots of different placements; some you will have enjoyed, some less so, but in all you had to be passed as competent. It is unlikely that you had much influence on where you were placed and you will have had to accept the range of experiences offered. So when you started applying for jobs towards the end of your training you would have been looking for your 'dream job'. This would probably have been in a placement similar to one you had actually experienced and where you had felt appreciated. It is also likely that you will have tried to remain with the trusts that you have encountered, rather than looking further afield, to limit the stress of change.

Local employers will have been familiar with the placement restrictions imposed on you as an about-to-qualify student, and so would have looked at your ongoing achievement record document and personal tutor reference rather than experience. Applying for a post six months after qualifying is different; you now have post-registration experience and are a 'valuable commodity'. You may consider the word 'commodity' odd, and feel that that, as a potential employee, the power rests with the employer, but this is not really the case. Employers need workers, as without them all organisations would cease to function. So you need to ensure that you project yourself as not just a worker, but as a very desirable commodity, that any organisation would be delighted to employ.

In the scenario, you are asked to complete an application form rather than send a CV; this is common practice in the NHS, but may not be the case in other situations. Clearly you must apply in the required way, whether it is a completed in-house form, a CV or an expression of interest with a supporting letter. Failure to do as requested will immediately condemn your application to the rubbish bin! No one wants to employ someone who cannot follow simple instructions.

Many texts are written on the skills of applying for jobs and so this chapter will only deal with this briefly, giving you some pointers, and will then return to the specifics of nursing applications.

Curriculum vitae

McGee (2001) writes about how a CV should not be static but reflect the position that you are applying for, and he categorises CVs under the headings chronological, functional and targeted. Most of us would have a CV of the chronological type, listing our experience in reverse order with our most recent experience first. This is the way it should run, because any future employer wants to know what you are doing now, rather than what you did at school. Similarly, your portfolio should not simply be a continuation of the one you started at 15, opening with a school certificate, as this does not give the right impression.

Always keep a copy of your CV, ideally electronically, with the dates of significant events, and update it regularly: what was once a key aspect of your job may well now be past experience. Updating personal information is important and is a vital tool for a quick response to a job application. Similarly, always keep a copy of the material you sent in application for a job; you need to remind yourself what you wrote, or what the panel might refer to if you are shortlisted for an interview.

McGee's functional CV has parallels with a skills profile and this is an area that will be discussed in relation to the scenario. A targeted CV will relate to a specific post and could also be seen as supporting information, providing a rationale as to why you are suitable for the post. Whatever type of CV you produce, make sure it is accurate, clearly typed with a good layout and no spelling errors. This is a document to make an impression so that the potential employer wants to meet you. If you are unlucky enough to have to complete a hand-written form, do a practice run on a photocopy first, and then use your tidiest handwriting, with no alterations. Many books address CV writing in great detail and demonstrate the dos and don'ts that writers must tackle. For example, they consider which verbs to use to describe your achievements or what adjectives provide a positive view. They will stress the importance of correct grammar, spelling and presentation, even so far as the type of paper and number of folds needed to get the CV in an envelope.

Returning to the scenario, do you feel that the staff nurse working on the intensive care unit is at a clear advantage over you, because you are working outside the NHS in a nursing home? Many students certainly do and have expressed their concerns that once they leave the NHS they will never 'get back in'. This is certainly not true, because future employers will be looking for transferable skills and positive attitudes, not like-for-like practice. Students erroneously believe that you need to have been noticed or worked in an area to be recruited.

Consider what a staff nurse working for six months in ITU in the trust might have learnt and want to 'sell' to a future employer:

- an understanding of the trust's philosophy;
- an understanding of the types of patients treated there and when they are moved elsewhere;
- competence in managing the equipment that provides life support to patients;
- nursing care in areas such as hygiene, pressure sore prevention and nutrition;
- drug therapy associated with complex illness;
- aspects of psychosocial care related to ITU patient experiences.

Do any of the above really demonstrate your capabilities for an A&E job any more than the following statements, written following a nursing home experience?

- an understanding of the philosophy of the home's parent organisation;
- an understanding of the types of patients admitted to the home;
- competence in managing patients with dementia;
- nursing care in areas such as hygiene, pressure sore prevention and nutrition;
- drug therapy associated with terminal illness;
- psychosocial care of patients with long-term health needs.

What are needed are qualities that are transferable and show an understanding that can be rolled out to other arenas. So writing these six statements in a more comprehensive and transferable way following experience in a nursing home or ITU might look like the following.

1. *Working within the organisation/trust has enabled me to consider how the unit's philosophy on patient dignity can be translated into practice with long-stay/ITU patients. The needs of the patients and their families have to be considered alongside the requirements of medical treatment. For example, the importance of dignity for*

patients who have lost their social skills, due to the dementia disease process, or for patients nursed in the mixed-sex ITU, with minimal privacy.

In this statement you are demonstrating how you have actually applied a theoretical concept to your client group, something which you would be able to continue doing in an A&E situation.

2. *The A&E experience is only part of a treatment regime for most patients and many will need community support or services in their home, once discharged. My ability to liaise with other members of the multi-disciplinary team in supporting a patient demonstrates transferable and relevant communication skills, resource management and leadership.*

3. *My ability to converse with confused patients is also a real asset which I learnt in ITU/the nursing home and would help me deal with A&E clients.*

The skills of dealing with grieving relatives and friends are again transferable to A&E, whether gained in a nursing home or in ITU. The knowledge, skills and attitudes associated with effective assessment are also transferable.

4. *The patients encountered in the nursing home may well be similar to those being admitted through A&E, and will require my skills of assessment in areas such as nutrition or mobility. As a nurse with ITU experience I am familiar with the equipment used in the assessment or resuscitation of severely ill patients.*

From your experience state how all aspects of the nursing process are met in the confines of the patient's environment. Being able to plan future care and identify good time management skills as well as effective resource management is always useful wherever this is learnt.

5. The safe administration and storage of medicines should apply wherever you work, whether in a nursing home or ITU. But the community experience can be linked to how you work with the pharmacy or the family to get medication in an appropriate form and on time into the patient, whereas the ITU experience may provide familiarity with a range of intravenous drug administration skills.

6. Dealing effectively with psychosocial issues associated with the patient and family is readily applicable to the A&E setting and learnt in any practice area.

This example should have helped you see how the most important thing about applying for any job is to see how you match the criteria that are being required. All texts on applying for posts will suggest that you need to illustrate how you have the skills, knowledge and attitudes to meet potential employers' requirements better than anyone else. So once you have sent your CV or application form in and are offered an interview, you will need to build on these aptitudes. Your application should have sold your strengths and may have been a little creative, but at interview you may well be asked to explain these strengths further, so never lie.

So you get that dream job and it's all you ever wanted. Is that enough, or can you progress your career? This is the typical situation facing many staff: they enjoy where they are working but know that they need to do something else. It is at this point that you need to consider where you might want to be in five or ten years' time and only you will know your dreams and aspirations.

Skills and career path

McGee (2001, p12) suggests we should always recognise our own strengths and weaknesses as these should influence our career pathway. You should assess your people skills, practical skills, communication skills, mental skills, problem-solving skills and creativity, and in doing so recognise where your strengths lie. This should help guide your career choices as these are your six skills set.

Activity 10.2   *Team working*

These are both typical interview questions, although they may be worded differently, so you need to think about them.

Think about the six skills sets described. Which would your best friend say are your strengths? Give a few examples.

You may also have a 'down side' which makes you less effective at work than you'd like to be. What are the skills you need to improve?

An outline answer is provided at the end of the chapter.

Most newly qualified nurses think they know the ideal job for them, and if they are lucky may be on a pathway leading there. For many of us the career path is more winding. Career 'detours' need not be a waste of your time; they can lead to a broadening of your horizons in ways you never considered. Do bear in mind that if you register by the age of 25 you are likely to have a working life of 40–45 years. So if you make a detour, forced or otherwise, you have to learn from it; you have to be able to reflect back (even on the bad experiences) and recognise how you have developed. You will have gained transferable skills, the same as those of your pre-registration programme, although some experiences can be even more painful when you are a qualified and registered practitioner.

There is never any harm in applying for a job that might seem slightly out of reach; you need to push yourself forward, and in this political and financial climate there will always be competition from others trying to sell themselves. You need to convince an employer that you have the skills and talent to do the job, even if you have a non-traditional background. If you don't believe in yourself, why should anyone else believe in you?

As a word of caution, not all job applications will result in success and this can be terribly disheartening. However, the most important aspect of rejection is the ability to maintain a belief in yourself and never give up trying. If you are rejected, try to get post-application feedback; it might help in the future.

Maintaining your career path

Maintaining your registration

If you decide to be a stay-at-home mum, or dad, you need to build that into your career planning. This is because it may well be important for you to maintain your registration while absent from full-time or continuous employment; otherwise the NMC will require you to follow a 'return to practice' programme after more than five years' absence. This will require studies and fees that may well cost considerable amounts, even assuming a programme is available locally. So, although it may be expensive to maintain registration and difficult to fulfil the NMC practice requirement, it may be worthwhile. In 2012 the requirement is to pay your annual fee with a minimum practice requirement of 100 hours of practice over five years (for nurses), plus evidence of continuous professional development (NMC, 2011). So remember, no matter how difficult this might be, returning to nursing or midwifery when your registration has lapsed may be even more difficult.

Enhanced Criminal Record Bureau (CRB)

Life does not always run smoothly and one problem that you may never have considered is criminality. One of the saddest things to happen to some staff and students is that they fall foul of the law in a fairly minor way; typically after a rather wild night out they accept a 'caution' for being drunk and disorderly. A caution means that you have accepted a criminal charge and this will always appear on an enhanced CRB check, it is never 'spent' in terms of the Rehabilitation of Offenders Act 1974 and subsequently the Independent Safeguarding Authority (Dimond, 2011). It is really important to remember that if you are asked to 'accept a caution' by the police, this has long-term implications and may not be the 'easiest option'.

If you do have any form of conviction you must declare it to a current employer and on any application form or at interview. Failure to do so is likely to be more damaging to your career than owning up to the problem when it is discovered by the employer, as it suggests dishonesty.

Social networking sites

Most of us use IT for communication more than pen and paper these days and sometimes we seem overwhelmed with electronic communication in the form of e-mail or text. The problem arises from the public nature of some types of communication such as Twitter or Facebook as these are accessible to anyone. So never put online material which you might later be embarrassed by or which would present you in an unfavourable light to an employer. Typical problem areas are the photograph of you in a revealing or drunken pose or a statement where you are critical of a named colleague, patient or organisation. You must remember that, once registered, you are always a nurse, so whatever you do, whether in work or outside, will reflect on your registration and hence your ability to practise. Also you might need to consider a new e-mail address to use in communication with employers, as one that is rather flippant or rude may not convey the right impression.

Post-registration education for professional practice (PREPP) (NMC, 2011)

The NMC rules identify that you must undertake a minimum of 35 hours of professional development every three years to ensure that you remain up to date. It is important to consider that mandatory annual training, as required by your employer, probably isn't included, although self-directed study would be. All registrants are required to maintain a portfolio which the NMC could ask to view when your annual registration fee is due.

Activity 10.3   *Communication*

Take time to review both your portfolio and CV. Your portfolio should be well presented and up to date without any irrelevant or out-of-date material. Look again at the style of your CV, and make sure it is available electronically.

No outline answer is given for this activity.

Future career development opportunities

Have you thought of the wealth of areas that your registration might lead to, or are you focused on your local NHS trust, where you know the staff and the policies? It is understandable that you might see your career there as long-term, but all too often circumstances make us rethink.

Activity 10.4   *Decision-making*

Ask yourself what would make you think about a change in job or employer.

An outline answer is provided at the end of the chapter.

Academic pathways

It is important in planning your career that you start to think about how hard you had to work to get your baseline registration; critically ask yourself how difficult intellectually it was to get your degree. Only you will know whether you were stretched academically to your limits or that you could have done more if you'd tried harder. This is not being critical, just asking you to be honest with yourself. Some qualified staff really struggle with further academic studies, whereas others flourish when the pressures are self-imposed. If you are considering further study, these are crucial questions.

The requirements of PREPP need you to continue with lifelong learning, not lifelong studying. Do not feel pressured into undertaking a course which you won't enjoy at least some of the time. There is nothing more disheartening than starting on a programme of study and being unable to complete it in a reasonable time.

Even if you don't want to become an academic, you will be required to support the learning of others, be they new members of staff, healthcare assistants or students, as dictated by the *Code of Conduct* (NMC, 2008b). The first stage of this is to undertake some form of mentorship training to support learners in practice, as this will help you understand what helps and what hinders learning. (Ideally, it should fit within a postgraduate framework and might eventually contribute to you studying for a Master's-level qualification.) Some mentors will continue to develop their teaching skills through qualifications that are recordable with the NMC as practice teacher or teacher (NMC, 2008a). You should be aware that not all nurse educators work in universities; many work within trusts as continuous professional development educators or as specialist skills trainers. If you see yourself in academia long-term you must work towards a Master's qualification or PhD.

Clinical pathways

Perhaps your strengths lie in clinical work, where you have a passion for a particular aspect of clinical nursing, usually identified around a medical condition. For instance, titles such as cystic fibrosis clinical nurse specialist, nurse consultant endoscopist or lead nurse dementia care indicate the development of nursing practice that overlaps with traditional medical expertise. These nurses have developed their knowledge through specialist training, research, publications and patient care and these roles are expanding. However, even the government recognises the importance of expert 'general' nurses, as it supports the modern matron role in ensuring the quality of care.

Outside the NHS, private hospitals and the care sector employ large numbers of staff in junior, senior, full- and part-time posts. All these roles or similar ones may be familiar to you, but what about nursing outside the usual care settings? Have you considered the role of nurses in the armed forces or as flight attendants for the acutely ill? A nursing qualification may in fact assist you in getting a post with an airline. Other nurses working in the UK are employed in the prison and police custody services, or working as specialists with medical equipment companies. Still more work with the leisure industry on cruise ships or travel further through employment in the Middle East, Australia or in non-governmental agencies. The world could be your oyster.

Remember, it doesn't matter if you don't have aspirations to climb the managerial or academic ladder; what you must do is strive to provide the best possible care to clients or patients in an a world of competing demands, whatever position you hold.

Scenario

Having enjoyed orthopaedics as a student nurse, you applied for a post in the directorate of a major teaching hospital and have been appointed. Six months later you decide to leave and get some varied experience, by working for three months as an agency nurse, going to other hospitals and specialities, including lots of gynaecology. Not being very imaginative, but not wanting ITU or midwifery, you are accepted on a renal and urology course full-time. You get married and after the course finishes follow your husband's job move; he is appointed to a more rural area and property is cheaper, so by mutual decision you leave your job. The only available post where he is based is in renal work, which you accept but eventually return to orthopaedics, and undertake studies in this area and now you want to teach. There are no teaching posts available so you undertake management and keep applying to teach; eventually you are accepted into orthopaedic teaching, but now love management as well. You undertake a range of courses in teaching and management, remarry, move home again and eventually buy a hotel, where you undertake more first aid and emergency treatment than in the rest of your nursing! And then you start writing books for nurses.

Activity 10.5 · Reflection

When you read this scenario, did you think it was chaotic or did you find it interesting? Would you want your career to mirror it or to be more structured?

As this is a personal reflection, no outline answer is supplied.

The scenario is of course a summary of the author's own career, which has been unstructured, unplanned but always interesting. Alas it never included travelling with the job, as colleagues have done. Maybe one day your fellow student group will have a 30-year reunion and you can compare the varied career paths you have had.

What will never change, wherever you work, is your attitude toward both patients and colleagues. You must always love caring for patients and clients with dignity and respect, whatever you do. Always behave toward colleagues the way you would like to be treated, and never forget how scary it is being a student or moving to a new job.

Activities: brief outline answers

Activity 10.1

You should have included areas such as

- increased knowledge of medicines management;
- ability to lead a team;
- ability to prioritise care needs;
- enhanced communication skills with the multidisciplinary team;
- resource management and financial issues.

Activity 10.2

Your strengths typically might be team player, honest, good at leading, good communicator, works hard, fun to be with.

The downside might be: not good at managing time, untidy, doesn't always think before speaking.

Activity 10.4

You might have replied:

- wanting promotion or more money or moving locality with family or partner;
- wanting to reduce hours or have a different work pattern or the opportunity to travel.

Further reading and useful websites

www.totaljobs.com/careers-advice/cvs-and-applications/application-forms-two

To read more about job applications.

www.nhsemployers.org/PlanningYourWorkforce/Pages/Planning-your-workforce.aspx

To read more about workforce planning in the NHS, including recruitment and workforce well-being.

www.nhscareers.nhs.uk/nursing.shtml

For more information on the variety of posts for nurses in the NHS.

References

Anaesthesia UK (2010) *The Laryngeal Mask*. www.frca.co.uk/article.aspx?articleid=238.

Bach, S and Ellis, P (2011) *Leadership, Management and Team Working*. Exeter: Learning Matters.

Beck, D and Srivastava, R (1991) Perceived level and sources of stress in baccalaureate nursing students. *Journal of Nursing Education*, 3: 127–33.

Benner, P (1982) From novice to expert. *American Journal of Nursing*, 82(3): 402–7.

Berne, E (1964) *The Games People Play: The psychology of human relationships*. New York: Ballantine Books.

Bishop, V (ed.) (2009) *Leadership for Nursing and Allied Health Care Professions*. Maidenhead: McGraw Hill/Open University Press.

Blake, R and Mouton, J (1985) *The New Managerial Grid 111: The key to leadership excellency*. Houston, TX: Gulf Publishing.

British Association of Day Surgery (2004) *Integrated Care Pathways for Day Surgery Patients*. www.daysurgery uk.net/bads/joomla/files/handbooks/IntegratedCarePathways.pdf.

Bryans, W (2005) *Resource Management in Health and Social Care: Essential checklists*. Oxford: Radcliffe.

Cass, H (2006) *The NHS Experience: The snakes and ladders' guide for patients and professionals*. London: Routledge.

Clinical Audit Support Centre (2011) www.clinicalauditsupport.com/what_is_clinical_audit.html.

Coates, V (1985) *Are they Being Served? An investigation into the nutritional care given by nurses to acute medical patients and the influence of ward organisational patterns on that care*. London: Royal College of Nursing.

Creed, F and Spiers, C (2010) *Care of the Acutely Ill Adult: An essential guide for nurses*. Oxford: Oxford University Press.

Department of Health (1993) *The Patient's Charter: Raising the standard*. London: HMSO.

Department of Health (1997) *The New NHS: Modern, Dependable*. webarchive.nationalarchives.gov.uk/+/www.dh.gov.uk/en/Publicationsandstatistics/Publications/PublicationsPolicyAndGuidance/DH_4008869.

Department of Health (1999) *Making a Difference: Strengthening the nursing, midwifery and health visitor contribution to health and healthcare: summary*. www.dh.gov.uk/en/Publicationsandstatistics/Publications/PublicationsPolicyAnd Guidance/DH_4007599.

Department of Health (2000a) *Comprehensive Critical Care: A review of adult critical care services*. London: Department of Health.

Department of Health (2000b) *An Organisation with a Memory*. London: HMSO.

Department of Health (2009) *Competencies for Recognising and Responding to Acutely Ill Adults in Hospital*. Draft guidelines for consultation. London: HMSO.

Department of Health (2010a) *Liberating the NHS: Developing the healthcare workforce. A consultation on proposals*. Leeds: Department of Health.

Department of Health (2010b) *Essence of Care*. www.dh.gov.uk/en/Publicationsandstatistics/Publications/PublicationsPolicyAndGuidance/DH_119969.

Dimond, B (2011) *Legal Aspects of Nursing*, 6th edition. Harlow: Prentice Hall.

Dougherty, L and Lister, S (eds) (2011) *The Royal Marsden Hospital Manual of Clinical Nursing Procedures*, 8th edition. http://www.royalmarsdenmanual.com/view/online.html

Downie, C and Basford, PE (2003) *Mentoring in Practice: A reader*. London: Greenwich University.

Duffy, K (2003) *Failing to Fail: A qualitative study of factors that influence the decision regarding assessment of students' competence in practice*. Glasgow: Caledonian University/NMC 2.

EU Commission (2000) *Commission Staff Working Paper: A memorandum on lifelong learning*. Brussels: EU Commission.

European Foundation (1997) *Preventing Absenteeism at the Workplace: Research summary*. ECU-34. Luxembourg: European Foundation for the Improvement of Living and Working Conditions.

General Medical Council (2012) www.gmc-uk.org/education/our_role_in_medical_education.asp.

Girvin, J (1998) *Leadership and Nursing: Essentials of Nursing Management*. London: Macmillan.

Glen, S and Wilkie, K (2000) *Problem-Based Learning in Nursing: A new model for a new context?* Basingstoke: Macmillan.

Goodman, B and Clemow, R (2008) *Nursing and Working with Other People*. Exeter: Learning Matters.

Hall, GM (ed.) (2007) *How to Present at Meetings*, 2nd edition. Oxford: BMJ Books/Blackwell.

Health and Safety Executive (2006) The development of a fatigue/risk index for shift workers. www.hse.gov.uk/research/rrpdf/rr446.pdf.

Healthcare Quality Improvement Partnership (2011) www.hqip.org.uk/.

Health Professions Council (2009) *Standards of Education and Training*. section 5 practice placement. London: Health Professions Council.

Hegyvary, ST (1982) *The Change to Primary Nursing: A cross-cultural view of professional nursing practice*. St Louis: Mosby.

Hersey, P and Blanchard, K (1989) Situational leadership grid, in Hersey, P, Blanchard, K and Johnson, DE (eds) *Management of Organizational Behavior: Utilizing human resources*, 5th edn. Englewood Cliffs, NJ: Prentice-Hall, p.117.

Honey, P and Mumford, A (1982) *Manual of Learning Styles*. London: Peter Honey Publications.

Kelemen, ML (2003) *Managing Quality*. London: Sage.

La Monica, E (1994) *Management in Health Care: A theoretical and experiential approach*. British adaptation by P Morgan. Hampshire: Macmillan.

La Monica Rigolosi, E (2005) *Management in Health Care: A theoretical and experiential approach*, 2nd edition. New York: Springer.

Learning Styles Questionnaire (2012) www.peterhoney.com/content/LearningStylesQuestionnaire.html.

Machiavelli, N (1515) translated by Marriott, WK (1908) www.constitution.org/mac/prince00.htm.

Marquis, B and Huston, C (1994) *Leadership Roles and Management Functions in Nursing: Theory and application*. Philadelphia, PA: Lippincott.

Marquis, B and Huston, C (2006) *Leadership Roles and Management Functions in Nursing: Theory and application*, 5th edition. Philadelphia, PA: Lippincott/Williams & Wilkins.

McGee, P (2001) *Write a Great CV ; Prepare a powerful CV that really works*. Oxford: How to Books.

McSherry, R and Pearce, P (2002) *Clinical Governance: A guide to implementation for healthcare professionals*. Oxford: Blackwell Scientific.

NHS (2004) *The NHS Knowledge and Skills Framework*. www.dh.gov.uk/publications.

NHS Choices (2010) *BMI Healthy Weight Calculator*. www.nhs.uk/Tools/Pages/Healthyweightcalculator. aspx.

NHS Executive (1998) *Working Time Regulations Implementation in the NHS*. Health Service circular 1998/204. London: HMSO.

NICE (2007) *Acutely Ill Patients in Hospital: Recognition of and response to acute illness in adults in hospital*. http:// publications.nice.org.uk/acutely-ill-patients-in-hospital-cg50.

NICE, CHI and RCN (2002) *Principles for Best Practice in Clinical Audit*. Abingdon: Radcliffe Medical Press.

Nursing and Midwifery Council (2004) *Quality Assurance* fact sheet c/2004. www.nmc-uk.org/Educators/ Quality-assurance-of-education/Factsheets/QA-Fact-sheet-C2004/.

Nursing and Midwifery Council (2007) British Council's International English Language Testing System (IELTS) requires pass at 7.0 from 9.0 in all papers. www.nmc-uk.org/Documents/Circulars/2007circulars/NM Ccircular01_2007.pdf.

Nursing and Midwifery Council (2008a) *Standards to Support Learning and Assessment in Practice*. www.nmc-uk. org/Documents/Standards/nmcStandardsToSupportLearningAndAssessmentInPractice.pdf.

Nursing and Midwifery Council (2008b) *Code of Conduct*. www.nmc-uk.org/code.

Nursing and Midwifery Council (2010) *Standards for Pre-registration Nursing Education*. London: NMC.

Nursing and Midwifery Council (2011) *The PREP Handbook*. www.nmc-uk.org/Documents/Standards/ NMC_Prep-handbook_2011.pdf.

Nursing Standard (2012) *Poor Quality Care Blamed on Workload*. nursingstandard.rcnpublishing.co.uk/news-and-opinion/analysis/poor-quality-care-blamed-on-workload/.

Porter-O'Grady, T (2003) A different age for leadership, part 1: new context, new content. *Journal of Nursing Administration*, 33(2): 105–10.

Powell, DJ and Brodsky, A (1998) *Clinical Supervision in Alcohol and Drug Abuse Counselling: Principles, models and methods*. San Francisco, CA: Jossey-Bass.

RapidBI (2007) http://rapidbi.com/swotanalysis/.

Sullivan, E and Decker, P (2009) *Effective Leadership and Management in Nursing*. Englewood Cliffs, NJ: Pearson Prentice Hall.

Talbot-Smith, A and Pollock, AM (2006) *The New NHS: A guide*. London: Routledge.

Tate, S and Sills, M (eds) (2004) *The Development of Critical Reflection in Health Professions*. Higher Education Academy Health Sciences and Practice Subject Centre. London: Kings College.

UK Parliament (2010) www.publications.parliament.uk/pa/cm201212/cmhansrd/cm120125/text/120 125w0001.htm.

Van Emden, J and Becker, L (2004) *Presentation Skills for Students*. Basingstoke: Palgrave Macmillan.

Vitello-Cicciu, J (2007) Emotional intelligence in the nursing profession. www.asrn.org/journal-nursing/ 202-emotional-intelligence-in-nursing-profession.html.

Watzlawick, P, Beavin-Bavelas, J and Jackson, D (1967) Some tentative axioms of communication. In: *Pragmatics of Human Communication – A study of interactional patterns, pathologies and paradoxes*. New York: WW Norton.

Woodhall, G and Stuttard, A (1999) *Financial Management: Essentials of nursing management series*. Basingstoke: Macmillan.

Working Time Regulations SI no 1833 (1998) www.legislation.gov.uk/uksi/1998/1833/contents/made.

Index

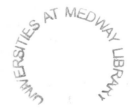